Musculoskeletal Imaging

Oxford Specialists Handbooks published and forthcoming

General Oxford Specialist Handbooks
A Resuscitation Room Guide
Addiction Medicine
Hypertension
Perioperative Medicine,
  Second Edition
Post-Operative Complications,
  Second edition
Pulmonary Hypertension

Renal Transplantation

Oxford Specialist Handbooks in Anaesthesia
Cardiac Anaesthesia
Day Case Surgery
General Thoracic Anaesthesia
Neuroanaethesia
Obstetric Anaesthesia
Paediatric Anaesthesia
Regional Anaesthesia,
Stimulation and Ultrasound Techniques

Oxford Specialist Handbooks in Cardiology
Adult Congenital Heart Disease
Cardiac Catheterization and Coronary
  Intervention
Cardiac Electrophysiology
Cardiovascular Magnetic Resonance
Echocardiography
Fetal Cardiology
Heart Failure
Nuclear Cardiology
Pacemakers and ICDs
Valvular Heart Disease

Oxford Specialist Handbooks in Critical Care
Advanced Respiratory Critical
  Care

Oxford Specialist Handbooks in End of Life Care
End of Life Care in Dementia
End of Life Care in Nephrology
End of Life in the Intensive
  Care Unit

Oxford Specialist Handbooks in Neurology
Epilepsy
Parkinson's Disease and Other Stroke
Medicine

Oxford Specialist Handbooks in Paediatrics
Paediatric Dermatology
Paediatric Endocrinology
  and Diabetes
Paediatric Gastroenterology, Hepatology,
and Nutrition
Paediatric Haematology
  and Oncology
Paediatric Intensive Care
Paediatric Nephrology
Paediatric Neurology
Paediatric Palliative Care
Paediatric Radiology
Paediatric Respiratory Medicine

Oxford Specialist Handbooks in Psychiatry
Child and Adolescent Psychiatry
Old Age Psychiatry

Oxford Specialist Handbooks in Radiology
Interventional Radiology
Musculoskeletal Imaging

Pulmonary Imaging

Oxford Specialist Handbooks in Surgery
Cardiothoracic Surgery
Colorectal Surgery
Hand Surgery
Liver and Pancreatobiliary Surgery
Operative Surgery, Second Edition
Oral Maxillofacial Surgery
Otolaryngology and Head and Neck Surgery
Paediatric Surgery
Plastic and Reconstructive Surgery
Surgical Oncology
Urological Surgery
Vascular Surgery

Oxford Specialist Handbooks in Radiology
Musculoskeletal Imaging

Edited by

Philip G. Conaghan

Professor of Musculoskeletal Medicine,
University of Leeds, Consultant Rheumatologist,
Leeds Teaching Hospitals NHS Trust and
Leeds Primary Care Trust, UK

Philip J. O'Connor

Consultant Musculoskeletal Radiologist,
Department of Clinical Radiology,
Leeds Teaching Hospitals Trust, UK

David A. Isenberg

ARC Diamond Jubilee Professor of Rheumatology,
Centre for Rheumatology,
Department of Medicine,
University College London, UK

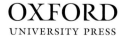

OXFORD
UNIVERSITY PRESS

OXFORD

UNIVERSITY PRESS

Great Clarendon Street, Oxford OX2 6DP

Oxford University Press is a department of the University of Oxford.
It furthers the University's objective of excellence in research, scholarship,
and education by publishing worldwide in

Oxford New York

Auckland Cape Town Dar es Salaam Hong Kong Karachi
Kuala Lumpur Madrid Melbourne Mexico City Nairobi
New Delhi Shanghai Taipei Toronto

With offices in

Argentina Austria Brazil Chile Czech Republic France Greece
Guatemala Hungary Italy Japan Poland Portugal Singapore
South Korea Switzerland Thailand Turkey Ukraine Vietnam

Oxford is a registered trade mark of Oxford University Press
in the UK and in certain other countries

Published in the United States
by Oxford University Press Inc., New York

British Library Cataloguing in Publication Data
Data available

Library of Congress Cataloging-in-Publication Data
Data available

Typeset by Cepha Imaging Private Ltd., Bangalore, India
Printed in China
on acid-free paper through
L.E.G.O. SpA—Lavis TN

ISBN 978–0–19–923577–3

10 9 8 7 6 5 4 3 2 1

Preface

The original concept of *Imaging in Rheumatology* was developed by myself and the late Peter Renton.

The book was well received but with the remarkable development of new imaging modalities producing images of ever-improving quality, it was agreed that a new edition of the book should reflect this and also be rather more interactive. Tragically, Peter died much too soon, but this volume has been co-edited with two outstanding colleagues, Philip G. Conaghan and Philip J. O'Connor. Together, we have attempted to produce an exciting, readable and well-informed volume that would be a genuine advance on the original volume. We would like to thank our contributors for (mostly!) keeping to the tight publishing schedule and hope that the reader will enjoy the breadth of topics covered, the quality of the images and the detailed information provided.

Finally, we would like to thank Susan Crowhurst from Oxford University Press, our often tough, but fair 'in-house' editor.

David A. Isenberg MD FRCP
ARC Diamond Jubilee Professor of Rheumatology,
Centre for Rheumatology,
Department of Medicine,
University College London

Contents

Detailed contents

Contributors

Nik Barnes
Radiology Department,
Royal Liverpool Children's
Hospital, UK
(Chapter 9 with Gavin Cleary)

Philip Bearcroft
Consultant Radiologist,
Addenbrooke's Hospital,
Cambridge University Hospitals
NHS Foundation Trust, UK
(Chapter 4 with Andrew Östör)

Robin Butler
Consultant Rheumatologist,
Robert Jones and Agnes Hunt
Orthopaedic Hospital NHS Trust,
Gobowen, Oswestry, UK
*(Chapter 8 with Radhesh K. Lalam
and Victor N. Cassar-Pullicino)*

Robert S.D. Campbell
Consultant Musculoskeletal
Radiologist,
Department of Radiology,
Royal Liverpool Hospital, UK

Victor N. Cassar-Pullicino
Radiology Department,
Robert Jones and Agnes Hunt
Orthopaedic Hospital NHS Trust,
Gobowen, Oswestry, UK
*(Chapter 8 with Robin Butler and
Radhesh K. Lalam)*

Gavin Cleary
Consultant Paediatric
Rheumatologist,
Alder Hey Children's NHS
Foundation Trust,
Liverpool, UK
(Chapter 9 with Nik Barnes)

Philip G. Conaghan
Professor of Musculoskeletal Medicine,
University of Leeds,
Consultant Rheumatologist,
Leeds Teaching Hospitals
NHS Trust and Leeds Primary
Care Trust, UK
(Chapter 2 with A.J. Grainger)

Joel David
Department of Rheumatology,
Nuffield Orthopaedic Centre,
Oxford, UK
*(Chapter 5 and 6 with Eugene
McNally, David Gay, and Voon Ong)*

David Elias
Department of Radiology,
Kings College Hospital NHS Trust,
London, UK
(Chapter 10 with David L. Scott)

David Gay
Radiology Department,
Nuffield Orthopaedic Centre,
Oxford, UK
*(Chapter 5 and 6 with Eugene
McNally, Joel David, and Voon Ong)*

Andrew J. Grainger
Consultant Musculoskeletal
Radiologist,
Chapel Allerton Orthopaedic
Centre, Leeds, UK
(Chapter 2 with Philip G. Conaghan)

Ian Griffiths
Consultant Rheumatologist and
Senior Clinical Lecturer,
Freeman Hospital,
Newcastle upon Tyne, UK
(Chapter 3 with Geoff Hide)

Philip Helliwell
Senior Lecturer in Rheumatology,
University of Leeds, UK
(Chapter 7 with Anthony Redmond and Philip Robinson)

Geoff Hide
Consultant Musculoskeletal
Radiologist,
Freeman Hospital,
Newcastle upon Tyne, UK
(Chapter 3 with Ian Griffiths)

David A. Isenberg
ARC Diamond Jubilee
Professor of Rheumatology,
University College London, UK
(Chapter 11 with Lynne Shand)

Radhesh K. Lalam
Radiology Department
Robert Jones and Agnes Hunt
Orthopaedic Hospital NHS Trust
Gobowen, Oswestry, UK
(Chapter 8 with Victor Cassar-Pullicino and Robin Butler)

Eugene McNally
Department of Radiology, Nuffield
Orthopaedic Centre, Oxford, UK
(Chapter 5 and 6 with David Gay, Joel David, and Voon Ong)

Tarnya Marshall
Consultant Rheumatologist,
Norfolk and Norwich University
NHS Trust, Norwich, Norfolk, UK
(Chapter 12 with Tom Marshall)

Tom Marshall
Consultant Radiologist,
Norfolk and Norwich University
NHS Trust, UK
(Chapter 12 with Tarnya Marshall)

Voon Ong
Senior Clinical Lecturer and
Honorary Consultant Rheumtologist
Centre for Rheumatology and
Connective Tissue Diseases, Royal
Free Hospital, London, UK
(Chapter 5 and 6 with David Gay, Eugene McNally and Joel David)

Andrew J.K. Östör
Consultant Rheumatologist and
Associate Lecturer
University of Cambridge
Director, Rheumatology Clinical
Research Unit
Addenbrooke's Hospital,
Cambridge University Hospitals
NHS Foundation Trust, UK
(Chapter 4 with Philip Bearcroft)

Anthony Redmond
Arthritis Research Campaign,
Senior Lecturer,
School of Medicine, University of
Leeds, UK
(Chapter 7 with Philip Helliwell and Philip Robinson)

Philip Robinson
Consultant Musculoskeletal
Radiologist,
Leeds Teaching Hospitals, UK
(Chapter 7 with Philip Helliwell and Anthony Redmond)

David L. Scott
Professor of Clinical
Rheumatology and Honorary
Consultant Rheumatologist
Kings College London School
of Medicine, UK
(Chapter 10 with David Elias)

Lynne Shand
Consultant Rheumatologist,
Aberdeen Royal Infirmary, UK
(Chapter 11 with David A. Isenberg)

Symbols and abbreviations

📖	cross reference
►	important
^{18}FDG	18 fluoro-deoxyglucose
ABCS	alignment, bones, cartilage and joints, soft tissues
AC	fibrocartilagenous acromioclavicular
ACL	anterior cruciate ligament
aCL	anticardiolipin
ANCA	anti-neutrophil cytoplasmic antibodies
AP	anteroposterior
aPL	antiphospholipid antibodies
APS	antiphospholipid syndrome
AS	ankylosing spondylitis
ATFL	anterior talo fibular ligament
ATP	adenosine triphosphate
AVN	avascular necrosis
AVN	avascular necrosis
BAL	bronchoalveolar lavage
BOOP	bronchiolitis obliterans organizing pneumonina
CDH	congenital dislocation of the hip
CFA	common femoral artery
CK	creatinine kinase
CNS	central nervous system
CPPD	calcium pyrophosphate dihydrate
CRITOL	capitellum, radial head, internal (medial) epicondyle, trochlea, olecranon, lateral epicondyle
CRP	C-reactive protein
CRPS	complex regional pain syndrome
CSF	cerebrospinal fluid
CSS	Churg–Strauss syndrome
CT	computed tomography
CTPA	computed tomography/pulmonary angiography
CTS	carpal tunnel syndrome
CXR	chest X-ray
DDH	developmental dysplasia of the hip
DEXA	dual energy X-ray absorptiometry

DHS	dynamic hip screw
DISH	diffuse idiopathic skeletal hyperostosis
DISI	dorsal intercalated segment instability
DM	dermatomyositis
DRU	distal radioulnar
DVT	deep vein thrombosis
EDTA	ethylenediaminetetraacetic acid
EMG	electromyogram
ENT	ear, nose and throat
ESR	erythrocyte sedimentation rate
FAI	femoroacetabular impingement
FDS	superficialis tendon
FHL	flexor hallucis longus
FOV	field of view
FPL	flexor pollicis longus
FS	fat saturated
GA	general anaesthetic
GCA	giant cell arteritis
GCT	giant cell tumour
GH	glenohumeral
GMAX	gluteus maximus
GMM	gluteus medius and minimus
GTPS	greater trochanteric pain syndrome
HIV	human immunodeficiency virus
HRCT	high resolution computed tomography
HSP	Henoch–Schönlein purpura
HU	Hounsfield Units
IBM	inclusion body myositis
IIM	Idiopathic inflammatory myopathies
IM	intermetatarsal
IP	iliopsoas
IPT	iliopsoas tendon
ITB	iliotibial band
iv	intravenous
IVC	inferior vena cava
IVD	intervertebral disc
JIA	juvenile idiopathic arthritis
LCL	lateral collateral ligament
MCL	medial collateral ligament
MCP	metacarpophalangeal

MDCT	multidetector row CT
MDP	methylene diphosphonate
MHC	major histocompatibility complex
MPA	microscopic polyangiitis
MPR	multiplanar reconstructed
MRA	magnetic resonance angiography
MRI	magnetic resonance imaging
MRS	magnetic resonance spectroscopy
MSK	musculoskeletal
MTO	metatarsophalangeal
NCS	nerve conduction studies
NEXUS	National Emergency X-Radiography Utilisation Study
NPSLE	Neuropsychiatric lupus
NSAIDs	non-steroidal anti-inflammatories
NSIP	non-specific interstitial pneumonia
NSIP	non-specific interstitial pneumonia
OA	osteoarthritis
OI	obturator internus
P31-MRS	phosphorus-31 MRS
PA	posteroanterior
PA	pulmonary angiography
PACS	patient archive and communication system
PAH	pulmonary arterial hypertension
PB	peroneus brevis
PCL	posterior cruciate ligament
PCr	phosphocreatine
PDE	phosphodiesters
PE	pulmonary embolus
PET	positron emission tomography
PFT	pulmonary function tests
Pi	inorganic phosphates
PIPJ	proximal interphalyngeal joint
PL	peroneus longus
PLL	posterior longitudinal ligament
PM	polymyositis
PME	phosphomonoesters
PSA	prostate specific antigen
PVNS	Pigmented villonodular synovitis
QF	quadratus femoris
RA	rheumatoid arthritis

RA	rheumatoid arthritis
RF	radio frequency
RF	rectus femoris
RI	resistance index
RS3PE	remitting seronegative symmetrical synovitis with pitting oedema
RSD	reflex sympathetic dystrophy
SA	sartorius
SBC	simple bone cysts
SCFE	slipped capital femoral epiphysis
SCIWORA	spinal cord injury without radiographic abnormality
SIJ	sacroiliac joint
SLAP	superior labral anterior–posterior
SLE	systemic lupus erythematosus
SPECT	single photon emission tomography
SRC	sceroderna renal crisis
SSC	systemic sclerosis
STIR	short TI inversion recovery
SVC	superior vena cava
TA	Takayasu's arteritis
TB	tuberculosis
Tc^{99}	$Technecium^{99}$
Tc-99m MIBI	technetium-99m sestamibi
TFCC	triangular fibro cartilage complex
TLCO	transfer factor of the lung for carbon monoxide
TNF	tumour necrosis factor
TOE	transoesophageal Doppler echocardiography
TOE	transoesophageal echo
TOP	transient regional osteoporosis
TR	repetition time
UCL	ulnar collateral ligament
UIP	usual interstitial pneumonia
US	ultrasound
V/Q	ventilation/perfusion
VISI	volar intercalated segment instability
WG	Wegener's granulomatosis

Chapter 1

How image modalities work

X-rays

- X-rays photons are a type of electromagnetic radiation, also referred to as ionising radiation.
- X–rays are produced from the tungsten anode of an X-ray tube when exposed to a stream of electrons emitted from a cathode through which is passed a very high voltage electrical current.
- Radiographic images are produced by passing an X-ray beam through body tissues. There is variable X-ray absorption by different bodily tissues. The transmitted X-rays interact with a detection device, such as photographic film.
- However, it is now common practice to utilize digital detection devices to create radiographic images to be viewed using computer monitors via a patient archive and communication system (PACS).
- Radiographs are 2D projectional images of the body in which all the anatomical structures are superimposed on each other.
- Anatomical structures are visualized as edges when tissues of different density lie adjacent to each other (e.g. bone against soft tissue).
- Radiographs can only display four different contrast densities:
  - Air
  - Fat
  - Soft tissue or fluid
  - Bone or calcification.
- Image resolution is dependant on the resolving power of the detecting device. Higher-resolution images require greater doses of ionizing radiation.
- In musculoskeletal (MSK) imaging radiographic images are often the first line investigation for demonstrating bone and joint abnormalities and areas of calcification. Soft tissue detail is very limited, although joint effusions may be demonstrated when fat pads are displaced by synovial fluid (e.g. elbow joint) (Fig 1.1).
- Radiographs are useful for:
  - Identification of fractures
  - Assessment of fracture healing
  - Localized bone pain
  - Arthritis
  - Bony deformity.
- Radiographs are of limited value when:
  - There is complex bony anatomy (e.g. spine, skull base etc.)
  - Demonstration of soft tissue structures is more important than identifying bony abnormalities (e.g. cartilage, ligaments etc.)
- Fluoroscopy is a means of producing real time moving X-ray images by using a continuous or pulsed X-ray beam and displaying the images on a TV monitor.
- Fluoroscopy is useful for guiding some interventional radiological procedures (e.g. spinal and joint injections or bone biopsy). It is also used in surgical theatres for orthopaedic operations requiring placement of implantable devices (e.g. joint prostheses) (Fig 1.2).

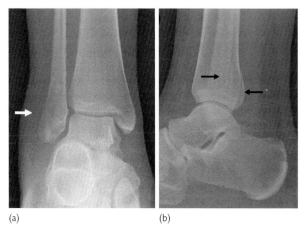

(a)   (b)

Fig. 1.1 (a) AP and (b) lateral radiographs of the ankle. Soft tissue swelling overlying the lateral aspect of the ankle (white arrow), is associated with fractures of the fibula and posterior tibia (black arrows). The fractures are barely visible on the AP view, which emphasises the importance of two-view radiography for trauma imaging.

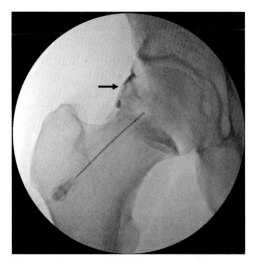

Fig. 1.2 Fluoroscopic X-ray image of the hip during an image guided injection of steroid. The needle is clearly visualized, and a small injection of iodinated contrast is visible (black arrow), which confirms the intra-articular location of the needle prior to injection.

Computed tomography

- Computed tomography (CT) is an X-ray-based technique that produces cross-sectional images of the body.
- Cross-sectional images differ from projectional images in that structures are not superimposed, and therefore provide more anatomical detail.
- In a CT scanner an X-ray tube is housed within a circular gantry surrounding a patient table. The X-ray tube rotates around the patient, continuously emitting an X-ray beam, while the patient moves through the scanner.
- Multiple rows of digital X-ray detectors are also housed within the CT gantry and detect the transmitted X-ray photons creating electrical signals. The CT image is constructed through a computerized process known as Fourier transformation.
- CT images can be viewed as 2D images in any orthoganal plane (axial, sagittal or coronal) or in multiple oblique planes (Fig 1.3). 3D images can also be obtained, usually with surface shading, although there are many post-processing techniques (Fig 1.4).
- Tissue density is presented as a grey scale image on a scale known as Hounsfield Units (HU), usually ranging from <−1000 to >+1000, with water set at 0 HU. Low-density structures such as air are dark or black, and high density bone is bright/white.
- Normal tissue densities include:
  - Air: −1000 HU
  - Lung: −700 ± 200 HU
  - Fat: −90 ± 10 HU
  - Parenchymal organs: +50 ± 40 HU
  - Muscle: +45 ± 5 HU
  - Trabecular bone: +130 ± 100 HU
  - Cortical bone: > +250 HU.
- The human eye can only differentiate about 20 different grey tones, so images have to be displayed as window levels, displaying tissues within a defined range of HU's (e.g. bone window, soft tissue window etc.). Image contrast is dependant upon the width of the window level.
- Although soft tissue contrast on CT is superior to radiographs, CT is inferior to MRI for delineation of most MSK soft tissue pathology.
- MSK CT is useful for:
  - Fractures of complex structures (e.g. spine)
  - Surgical planning for fracture fixation (e.g. calcaneal fractures)
  - Assessing fracture non-union or mal-union
  - Characterizing bone lesions to look for patterns of bone formation and bone loss
  - Identifying small joint loose bodies.
- Intravenous contrast is used much less frequently in MSK CT imaging than in chest/abdomen CT imaging. However, contrast may be administered into joints (CT arthrography) to identify intra-articular osteochondral abnormalities or into sinuses (CT sinography) to outline sinus tracks and bone/joint involvement.

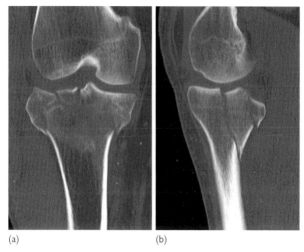

(a)   (b)

Fig. 1.3 Coronal (a) and sagittal (b) multiplanar reconstructed (MPR) CT images of a patient with a bicondylar, comminuted fracture of the proximal tibia. The 2D MPR images optimally demonstrate the degree of displacement of the fracture fragments and assist surgical planning.

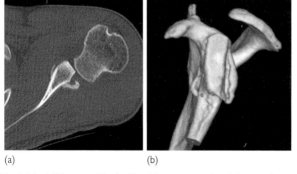

(a)   (b)

Fig. 1.4 Axial CT images of the shoulder; (a) in a patient with multidirectional traumatic instability. There are bony glenoid rim defects and anterior and posterior Hill–Sachs defects of the proximal humerus. The 3D surface shaded reconstruction of the scapula (b) with removal of the other bony structures shows the glenoid in profile and provides an excellent overview of the extent of bone loss.

Nuclear medicine: scintigraphy

- In MSK imaging the common scintigraphic examinations include:
  - Isotope bone scans
  - Isotope labelled white cell scans or Leucoscans.
- Scintigraphy involves an intravenous (iv) injection of a radioactive isotope with a short half-life, most commonly Technecium[99] (Tc[99]) which emits gamma radiation.
- In the case of an isotope bone scan the Tc[99] is labelled with a compound which will attach to bone such as methylene diphosphonate (MDP bone scan).
- Images are acquired by the use of a gamma camera, which detects the emitted radiation from the patient.
- Images can be produced as a 2D planar projectional scan. Alternatively cross-sectional imaging using single photon emission tomography (SPECT) can be preformed to improve spatial resolution. In this case the gamma camera revolves round the patient producing images in a method analogous to CT imaging.
- Tc[99] MDP attaches to bone in areas of osteoblastic activity. Therefore the normal skeleton demonstrates a low level of uptake. However, avid uptake is seen in lesions such as fractures and metastases where osteoblastic activity is pronounced. Osteoclastic areas or avascular bone will be shown as areas devoid of uptake (photopaenic) (Fig 1.5).
- The indications for isotope bone scans have greatly reduced over recent years with increasing use of MRI, but has the advantage of visualizing the whole skeleton.

Isotope bone scans are useful for:
- Bony metastatic bone disease
- Stress and insufficiency fractures
- Acute osteomyelitis
- Metabolic bone disease and Paget's disease
- In the presence of orthopaedic metalwork which degrades MR images or if there are contraindications to MRI.

Indium[111] labelled white cell scans or Leucoscans (Tc[99] Sulesomab—a monoclonal antibody fragment), are more specific for bone infection than Tc[99] MDP bone scan.

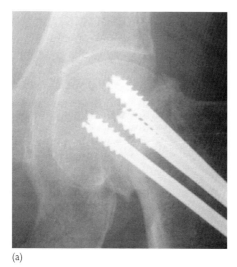

(a)

(b)

Fig. 1.5 Radiograph of the hip (a) following cannulated screw fixation for a fractured neck of femur. The isotope bone scan (b) demonstrates normal bony uptake in most of the bony structures. There is a linear area of increased uptake across the femoral neck (long black arrow) which represents the healing fracture line. However, there is also a photopaenic area within the superior aspect of the femoral head (short black arrow) which is due to early avascular necrosis, and which is not appreciated on the radiograph.

Nuclear medicine: positron emission tomography

Positron emission tomography (PET) involves an iv injection of a short-acting radioactive isotope that emits positrons, labelled to compounds that are normally used within the body such as glucose. A typical example is [18] fluoro-deoxyglucose ([18]FDG)

The positrons annihilate with electrons to produce 2 gamma rays which are emitted in opposite directions. Spatial location is determined by coincident detection of photon pairs.

PET scanners may be combined with CT (PET–CT) to provide fused images which give both the high spatial resolution of CT and the physiological data from PET (Fig 1.6).

The indications for PET–CT in MSK is very limited at present, and mostly involves oncology staging of bone metastases in oesophageal carcinoma, colorectal carcinoma, non-small cell lung carcinoma, lymphoma, melanoma etc. There are emerging roles for its use in bone and soft issue sarcoma.

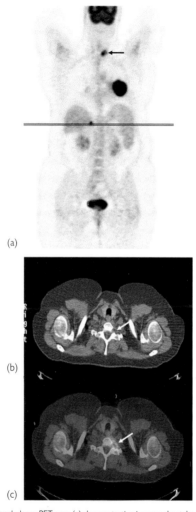

(a)

(b)

(c)

Fig. 1.6 Coronal planar PET scan (a) demonstrating increased uptake in the left hemithorax due to a lung carcinoma. There are also foci of uptake in the right adrenal and the in the left cervical region (black arrow). The axial CT image (b) shows a lytic lesion in the left C6 pedicle, which on the fused PET–CT image (c) corresponds to the area of abnormal uptake (white arrows), confirming the diagnosis of a bony metastasis.

Ultrasound

- Ultrasound (US) utilizes high-frequency sound waves to produce images of soft tissue structures.
- US waves are produced by stimulation of piezo-electric crystals by small electrical currents within the US probe.
- The US waves are transmitted from the US probe into the soft tissues and requires the use of a coupling gel on the skin surface.
- At soft tissue interfaces, some of the US beam is reflected back to the US probe. The reflected US waves in turn induce the peizo-electric crystals in the US probe to create electric currents which are the basis of the US signal.
- Image resolution is primarily influenced by the frequency of the US beam (higher frequencies can resolve narrower interfaces), and the width of the US beam.
- Soft tissue structures have variable degrees of acoustic impedance. Dense structures will attenuate the US beam rapidly, and this is more pronounced with higher-frequency US waves. Therefore deeper structures may need to be evaluated with lower-frequency probes, which results in lower image resolution.
- Very dense structures such as bone and calcification will reflect all the US waves, and acoustic shadowing is seen deep to the bone surface. US is therefore limited to assessment of the bone surface. A similar appearance is seen with air, which is a very poor conductor of US waves.
- Fluid has a very low acoustic impedance and will transmit all the US beam, and therefore lesions such as cysts will appear dark with no internal structures.
- Visualization of soft structures is not only dependent on the differences in acoustic impedance, but also the organization of the connective tissues. For example ligaments and tendons have very organized layers of collagen tissues which demonstrate multiple echo-bright parallel bright interfaces, when compared to adjacent fat which has less organized internal structure (Fig 1.7).
- Vascularity of tissues can be assessed using Doppler imaging (Fig 1.8). US also has the advantage of dynamic assessment, by passively or actively moving extremities throughout a range of movements, which cam improve delineation of defects in muscles, tendons and ligaments.
- US is useful for:
  - Assessment of tendons, ligaments and muscle disorders
  - Superficial soft tissue masses
  - Identification of joint effusions and synovitis
  - Guiding soft-tissue injection, aspiration and biopsy.

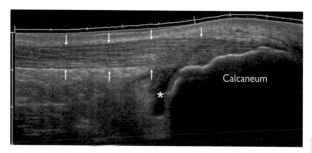

Fig. 1.7 Longitudinal US image of the distal Achilles tendon. The superficial and deep surfaces of the tendon (white arrows) are clearly distinguished from the surrounding fat tissues. Internal structure within the tendon is evident as parallel bands of hyper-reflective collagen bundle interfaces. The tendon insertion on the calcaneum can be seen, with acoustic shadowing deep to the bone surface. There is some fluid in the retro-calcaneal bursa (asterisk).

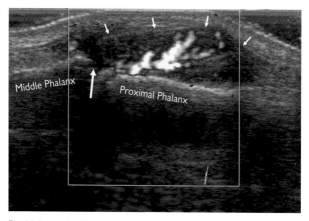

Fig. 1.8 Longitudinal Doppler US image of the proximal interphalyngeal (PIP) joint (long white arrow) of the finger in a patient with rheumatoid arthritis. An area of hypo-reflective active synovitis is seen arising from the joint (small white arrows), with prominent internal vascularity. The hyper-reflective surface of the phalanges is clearly evident.

Magnetic resonance imaging

- MR images are created by utilising the interaction between unbound hydrogen protons within the body and strong magnetic fields (typically 1.0–3.0 Tesla).
- Protons have a magnetic dipole moment, and align with the main magnetic field of the MR scanner.
- Other magnetic fields known as radio frequency (RF) pulses are applied at different angles to the main magnetic field creating a change in the alignment of the protons.
- When the RF pulse is turned off the protons realign with the main magnetic field by processes known as T1 and T2 relaxation times.
- These relaxation processes induce electrical currents within receiver coils which forms the basis of the MR signal from which images are generated.
- Spatial location is generated by using variable gradient RF coils in the x, y and z directions which in turn varies the strength of the electrical currents induced in the receiver coils.
- Different body tissues have variable densities of unbound protons, and variable T1 and T2 relaxation times.
- Pulse sequences are designed to generate images from the induced signal in the receiver coils that are relatively weighted to T1 relaxation, T2 relaxation or proton density. Sequences designed to reduce signal from fat tissues are known as fat-saturated images (e.g. STIR images), and can help improve lesion conspicuity.
- MR images are presented as grey scale images with low signal intensity (SI) tissue as dark, and high SI tissues as bright. One of the main differences between T1W and T2W images is the SI of fluid (T1W, low to intermediate SI; T2W, high SI) (Fig 1.9). Bone cortex is low SI intensity on all pulse sequences due to the lack of unbound hydrogen protons.
- Image Contrast is dependent on many factors including:
  - Intrinsic factors
    - T1 and T2 relaxation times
    - Proton density
  - Extrinsic factors:
    - Parameters of pulse sequence: e.g. repetition time (TR) between RF pulses.
- MRI is useful for:
  - Spinal imaging
  - Internal derangement of joints
  - Primary soft tissue and bone tumours
  - Acute and chronic soft issue injuries to tendons, ligaments and muscle
  - Osteomyelitis and soft tissue infection.

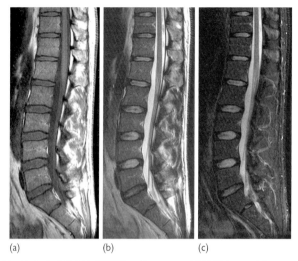

(a)   (b)   (c)

Fig. 1.9 Sagittal T1W (a), T2W (b) and fat-suppressed STIR (c) images of the lumbar spine. The cerebrospinal fluid (CSF) around the cauda equina, and the intervertebral discs on the T1W images are low to intermediate SI (dark), but high SI on the T2W and STIR images. Subcutaneous fat tissue is high SI on the TW and T2W images but low SI on the STIR images. The fatty marrow of the vertebral bodies is also lower SI on the STIR images than on the T1W and T2W images.

- IV contrast (Gadolinium) may be administered to help differentiate areas of inflammatory change from fluid, or viable and non-viable tumour. Intra-articular contrast (MR arthrography) is frequently used for internal derangement of some large joints to assess cartilage and ligaments (Fig 1.10).

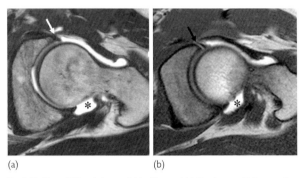

(a)   (b)

Fig. 1.10 Normal (a) and abnormal (b) oblique axial MR arthrographic images of the hip in two different patients. The joint recesses are filled with high SI intensity intra-articular contrast (asterisks). The normal fibro-cartilaginous labrum is seen as low SI triangular area at the bony margin of the acetabulum (white arrow). In (b) contrast undercuts the base of the labrum (black arrow) which indicates the presence of a labral tear or detachment.

Part 1

Investigations by anatomical region

Investigating knee region problems

Anatomy

The normal knee joint comprises two tibio-femoral compartments and a patello-femoral compartment. The articulating surface of each bone is lined with hyaline cartilage.

The knee joint also contains two hemicircular fibrocartilage menisci in the medial and lateral compartments.

The patella lies anteriorly with the quadriceps tendon attaching to its upper pole and the patellar tendon below. A number of bursae are located in the anterior compartment of the knee.

Knee stability is maintained by the surrounding musculature along with four major ligaments and associated capsular tissues. The ligaments are:

- the medial and lateral collateral ligaments
- the anterior cruciate ligament (ACL) which runs from the lateral side of the intercondylar notch posteriorly to the anterior attachment on the tibial plateau adjacent to the tibial spines
- the posterior cruciate ligament (PCL) originating from the medial femoral condyle and inserting onto the posterior aspect of the central tibial plateau.

Posteriorly, the popliteal fossa contains the hamstring muscles, the popliteal artery and nerves. Three hamstring muscles are identified. The laterally located biceps femoris, inserting as a tendon into the fibular head, the semimembranosus which has a complex tendon insertion into the posteromedial joint capsule as well as the tibia and femur, and the semitendinosus tendon which inserts into the medial tibia. Along with the gracilis and sartorius tendons the semitendinosus tendon forms the pes anserinus at its insertion. A bursa is associated with this insertion.

The non-articulating intra-articular surfaces of the joint are lined with synovium.

Imaging modalities
Radiography
- Bony structures
- Joint space changes seen in arthritis
- Calcified loose bodies
- Some soft tissue changes, including thickening of the suprapatellar pouch (stripe) due to fluid or synovitis

Magnetic resonance imaging (MRI)
- Bone marrow changes
- Internal knee structures including the menisci, ligaments, and articular cartilage
- Loose bodies
- Soft tissue masses and cysts

▶MRI is relatively insensitive to subtle bone avulsions.

Ultrasound (US)
- Superficial soft tissue structures such as the patellar and quadriceps tendon, and the collateral ligaments
- Soft tissue masses
- Joint fluid and synovitis

US is also useful for guiding interventional procedures
▶US does not 'see through' bone. Bone marrow is not visualized and structures hidden by overlying bone will not be visualized. Consequently US is not helpful for showing the cruciate ligaments or menisci.

Computed tomography (CT)
- Fine bone detail
- CT is the imaging modality of choice for subtle fractures and understanding the 3D configuration of fractures

Anterior cruciate ligament

Clinical features

Tears of the anterior cruciate ligament are not uncommon after significant trauma, such as in sportsmen. A story of acute injury with immediate swelling (even within 1 hour) is suggestive of significant trauma to the ACL. People may hear an audible popping sound.

The other major presenting feature of an ACL tear, especially in the chronic situation, is knee instability which may be worse with rotational lateral movements.

Examination findings include a positive Lachman's test and/or a positive anterior drawer sign, and increased hyperextension of the affected knee compared to the other side.

ACL tears are commonly associated with medial meniscus damage.

The major long-term concern is premature osteoarthritis. It is interesting that large cohort studies show quite a high frequency of previously unknown ACL tears, including complete tears, suggesting that injury of these ligaments may often go undiagnosed.

Imaging modalities

Radiography

Plain radiography may be normal or demonstrate evidence of:
- an effusion
- an avulsion fracture. Classically a Segond fracture is seen, representing avulsion of capsular tissues from the anterolateral tibial plateau. When seen it is highly specific for an ACL injury. Fig. 2.1 shows an AP knee radiograph demonstrating a segond fracture (arrow) in a patient with an ACL tear.

Magnetic resonance imaging (MRI)

MRI demonstrates:
- ligament discontinuity. Fig. 2.2a demonstrates an ACL tear with complete disruption of the ACL with high-signal fluid interposed between the torn fibres (*).
- an abnormal course to the ACL. On the sagittal image the ligament should parallel the roof of the intercondylar notch. In Fig. 2.2a the anterior margin of the ligament (arrow) appears to sag away from the intercondylar notch roof (arrowhead).
- abnormal signal within the ligament (best evaluated on coronal and axial imaging)
- lateral compartment bone bruising in the acute situation as a result of impaction between the bones at the time of injury reflecting the mechanism involved (pivot shift). Fig. 2.2b shows marrow oedema in the weight-bearing medial femoral condyle (arrow). A corresponding bone bruise was also seen posteriorly in the lateral tibial plateau.
- a joint effusion/haemarthrosis
- an associated meniscal tear

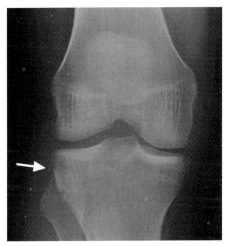

Fig. 2.1 AP knee radiograph demonstrating a segond fracture (arrow) in a patient with an ACL tear. The anterior margin of the ligament (arrow) appears to sag away from the intercondylar notch roof (arrowhead).

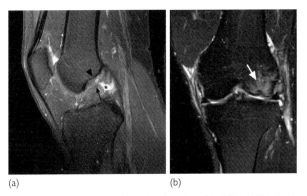

(a)   (b)

Fig. 2.2 (a) and (b) ACL tear with complete disruption of the ACL with high-signal fluid interposed between the torn fibres (*). The anterior margin of the ligament (arrow) appears to sag away from the intercondylar notch roof (arrowhead). 2.2 (b) shows marrow oedema in the weight-bearing medial femoral condyle (arrow). A corresponding bone bruise was also seen posteriorly in the lateral tibial plateau.

Posterior cruciate ligament

Clinical features

Injuries to the PCL are much less common than to the ACL due to its greater strength. The usual mechanism of injury is posterior translation of the tibia in the flexed knee and this most frequently occurs in motor vehicle accidents (dashboard trauma) and sporting injuries. People may complain of instability, although this may be minor if the ACL is still intact. The major long-term concern is premature osteoarthritis and patellar tendinopathies.

Examination findings include a visual sag (with knee in 90° of flexion and patient lying supine) and a positive posterior drawer test.

Imaging modalities

Radiography

Plain radiographs may demonstrate:

- an avulsion fracture. This typically occurs from the fibular styloid and when seen is highly predictive of a PCL tear.

Magnetic resonance imaging (MRI)

MRI may demonstrate:

- discontinuity of the ligament. Fig. 2.3 shows a PCL tear with the ligament seen to be discontinuous (arrow) ending abruptly as a result of a distal tear
- increased signal within the ligament. The normal ligament is of low signal on all sequences.
- Bone bruising of the anterior aspect of the lateral tibial plateau and weight-bearing aspect of the lateral femoral condyle may be seen as a result of impaction between the bones sustained at the time of injury reflecting the mechanism involved
- an associated ACL or collateral ligament disruption or meniscal tear

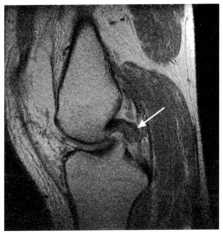

Fig. 2.3 PCL tear. The ligament is seen to be discontinuous (arrow) ending abruptly as a result of distal tear.

Menisci

Clinical features

Meniscal tears may be asymptomatic or present with intermittent pain and focal swelling. Pain on rotational movement of the knee (perhaps related to the location of the tear) may be present.

▶ Reported 'locking' of the knee is relatively uncommon but a good indication of a meniscal tear or loose body in the knee joint. However, locking should be distinguished from 'gelling' which is extremely common in osteoarthritic knees and refers to the prolonged pain/stiffness in the joint after a period of inactivity such as sitting or kneeling without moving.

▶ A report of the knee 'giving way' that is not related to acute trauma usually suggests weak quadriceps muscles and is sometimes an instantaneous reaction to acute pain. Only occasionally does it signify meniscal locking or ligament tears.

Examination findings of a torn meniscus may include tenderness along the relevant joint line and a positive McMurray's test; there may also be pain on forced hyperextension of the knee.

Imaging modalities

Radiography

Plain radiographs are usually normal, although if a meniscal tear is long-standing secondary osteoarthritis change may be seen.

Magnetic resonance imaging (MRI)

The cardinal features of a meniscal tear on MRI are:

- Abnormal increased signal within a meniscus extending to one or both articular surfaces of the meniscus. The normal meniscus shows low signal on all sequences. Fig. 2.4 shows a tear of the posterior horn of the medial meniscus. High signal is seen within the posterior horn extending to both inferior and superior surfaces (arrow). The normal anterior horn is also seen (arrow head).
- Alteration in the normal meniscal morphology
- Displacement of a meniscal fragment or flap

▶ although the normal meniscus shows low signal on all sequences myxoid degeneration will be seen as increased signal. However, this is typically non-linear in configuration and will not extend to an articular surface.

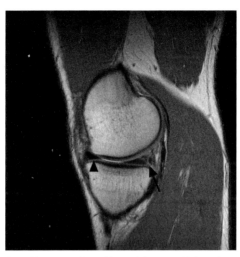

Fig. 2.4 Tear of the posterior horn of the medial meniscus. High signal is seen within the posterior horn extending to both inferior and superior surfaces (arrow). The normal anterior horn is also seen (arrowhead).

Meniscal cysts

Clinical features

Meniscal tears may be associated with meniscal cyst formation. Such cysts are relatively uncommon but when seen present as a mass lesion or swelling in the joint line. They communicate with the meniscal tear, but may dissect through the periarticular soft tissues over some distance so the bulk of the cyst lies remotely from the site of communication. Patients may complain of a tender swelling lying on the joint margin. There may be a history of previous knee injury.

Earlier literature would suggest that meniscal cysts more frequently arise from the lateral meniscus. MRI studies now suggest that they are seen medially and laterally with equal prevalence. However, the broad medial collateral ligament and other medial capsular structures tend to retain the medial cysts reducing the incidence of their clinical presentation.

Examination findings will include a local tender swelling (may be soft of firm to compression) with or without associated meniscal findings.

Imaging modalities

Radiography

Plain radiographs may demonstrate a soft tissue mass adjacent to the knee joint which may occasionally erode adjacent bone.

Magnetic resonance imaging (MRI)

- A cystic collection of fluid, often multiloculated, communicating with a meniscal tear. Fig. 2.5 shows a cyst in the medial joint line (arrow) which communicates with the meniscus (arrowhead). A tear was shown within the body of the meniscus.

Differential diagnosis includes:

- Bursae and synovial cysts communicating with the joint
  (will not communicate with the meniscal tear)
- Periarticular ganglion cysts

Other imaging modalities

- Although meniscal cysts are readily seen on ultrasound and a meniscal tear may be seen if it extends to the periphery of the meniscus, ultrasound is generally not useful for assessing the meniscus. However, it does remain a useful first line modality for assessing soft tissue mass lesions about the knee.

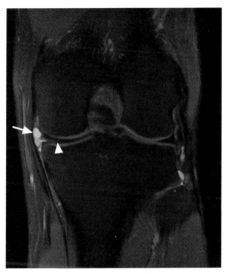

Fig. 2.5 Meniscal cyst in the medial joint line (arrow). The cyst communicates with the meniscus (arrowhead). A tear was shown in the body of the meniscus.

Tibio-femoral arthritis

Clinical features

The majority of problems in this area relate to osteoarthritis (OA). Typical clinical features of tibio-femoral osteoarthritis of the knee include:

- Less than 30min of morning stiffness (more than 60min suggests screen for inflammatory arthritis)

▶ Always distinguish gelling (inability to straighten knee after prolonged immobility such as kneeling or sitting) from true mechanical blocking which usually happens intermittently in gait, and which would suggest meniscal pathology.

- Pain may be predominantly medial and/or lateral and/or diffuse
- Pain increased with prolonged weight-bearing
- Occasional sensations of grating and grinding

Tibiofemoral osteoarthritis is commonly associated with patellofemoral involvement.

Imaging modalities

Radiography

Typical findings of tibiofemoral OA include:

- Reduced tibiofemoral joint space. Fig. 2.6a shows joint space loss in the medial compartment on this weight-bearing AP film

▶ Tibio-femoral views should always be weight-bearing in trying to assess severity of joint space narrowing. Remember that meniscal damage and extrusion can also contribute to apparent joint space loss.

- Marginal osteophytes (Fig. 2.6a arrow)
- Subchondral sclerosis and cyst formation
- Possible soft tissue swelling, reflecting synovial involvement or effusion
- Chondrocalcinosis
- Some degree of varus or valgus malalignment

Magnetic resonance imaging (MRI)

MRI findings in osteoarthritis are much more abundant than radiographic pathology:

- Cartilage loss—this can be focal or diffuse, partial or full thickness, or just demonstrate abnormal signal characteristics. Fig. 2.6b shows a coronal MRI scan from a patient with severe knee OA. There is complete loss of articular cartilage over the medial tibial plateau and femoral condyle (arrowheads).
- Osteophytes—these are often more extensive than seen on radiographs (Fig. 2.6b arrowhead).
- Bone marrow oedema
- Bone marrow cysts—these may occur in areas of bone marrow oedema
- Meniscal damage (tears and degeneration) and extrusion
- Synovitis (Fig. 2.6b asterix)

▶ Most routine MRI scans will not employ contrast agent and are not optimized for synovitis detection. Remember that the presence of synovitis is extremely common in osteoarthritis and in itself not indicative of an inflammatory arthritis.

Other differential diagnoses for synovial swellings include synovial lipomata, synovial chondromatosis or pigmented villonodular synovitis, all of which have characteristic MRI appearances.

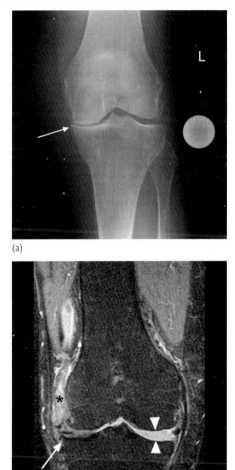

(a)

(b)

Fig. 2.6 (a) and (b) Tibiofemoral osteoarthritis. There is joint space loss in the medial compartment on the weight-bearing AP film (a). Osteophytes are also seen (arrow). (b) shown as MRI scan from a different patient. There is complete loss of articular cartilage over the medial tibial plateau and femoral condyle (arrowheads). Osteophyte (arrow) and synovitis (*) are also seen.

Other imaging modalities

Ultrasonography is useful for examining the medial and lateral ligaments, assessing the synovial cavity (medial and lateral recesses and suprapatellar pouch), and assessing periarticular swellings.

Loose bodies

They are most frequently seen as a result of osteoarthritis where cartilage or bone fragments become free-floating within the knee. The site of origin for these is not always evident.   Osteochondral loose bodies may also result from acute osteochondral injuries.

- Plain films may show a loose body if it contains sufficient calcification. Fig. 2.7a shows a small calcified loose body in the suprapatellar pouch on this AP knee radiograph.
- MRI readily demonstrates bone and cartilage loose bodies. Fig. 2.7b is a coronal MRI and shows the same patient as 2.7a. This shows the same loose body (arrow) but shows the body to be larger than appreci-ated on the plain film. The bulk of the body is cartilage (not seen on conventional film) with only a thin slither of bone seen along the deep surface of the body (lower signal). The body has moved more inferiorly between the time of the X-ray and the MRI.

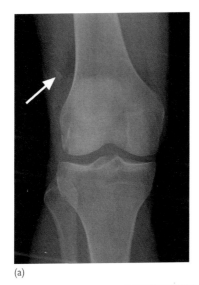

(a)

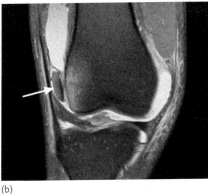

(b)

Fig. 2.7 (a) shows a small ossific loose body in the suprapatellar pouch (arrow). In (b) the same loose body is seen to be much larger because it is predominantly cartilaginous (arrow).

Patellofemoral arthritis

Clinical features

Patellofemoral joint pain is very common. Consider two groups:

- In younger females this is often called anterior knee pain and may be due to multiple biomechanical factors (e.g. poor muscle control, patella position). In particular this may be associated with hypermobility in other joints.
- Osteoarthritis is the commonest cause of patellofemoral pain in the over-50s.

▶ True patella pain (often felt 'behind the knee cap') needs to be distinguished from infra-patella pain (ligament or bursal problems).

Symptoms to suggest patello-femoral involvement may include pain on kneeling, pain on walking up and (especially) down stairs or slopes, or on getting out of chairs.

On examination there may be tenderness on compression of the patella onto the knee joint, or pain and crepitus on repeated flexion/extension of the knee.

Imaging modalities

Radiography

It is important to have adequate views of the patello-femoral joint; common views include the lateral knee and skyline views.

In cases of anterior knee pain without significant arthritis X-rays may be normal. Even with significant cartilage loss non-weight-bearing skyline and lateral views may be normal. In more advanced osteoarthritis osteophyte formation along with the typical subchondral changes of sclerosis, attrition, and cyst formation may be seen.

In the younger patient there may be clues to tracking abnormalities such as a high-lying patella (patella alta) or dysplasia of the femoral trochlea.

Magnetic resonance imaging (MRI)

The tomographic nature of MRI makes it well suited to examining the patello-femoral joint. As with plain films morphological abnormalities giving rise to maltracking may be seen in the form of trochlea dysplasia or a patellar alta. However, it is also possible to examine the patello-femoral joint dynamically looking for maltracking.

The articular cartilage of the patella is the thickest hyaline cartilage in the body and readily assessed with MRI. The earliest changes to articular cartilage seen are:

- Surface fibrillation
- Changes in signal within the cartilage substance

More significant cartilage damage may be seen in the form of cartilage tears and defects. Fig. 2.8 shows a full-thickness defect in the articular cartilage of the medial patella facet. Contrast the appearance with the normal cartilage seen in the lateral facet.

In the case of osteoarthritis MRI will show the typical changes previously described.

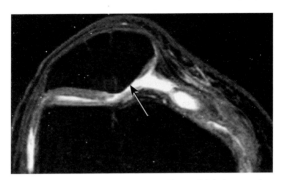

Fig. 2.8 MRI in a patient with anterior knee pain. There is full thickness cartilage loss over the medial patella facet (arrow).

Medial collateral ligament

Clinical features

Sporting injuries are probably the commonest cause for medial collateral ligament (MCL) damage, especially with forced valgus stress, e.g. a contact injury involving a blow to the lateral side of knee.

These injuries are painful with predominantly medial pain and often swelling. This pain is worse with any rotational stress.

On examination, valgus stress is painful and there may be limitation of both flexion and extension due to pain. Tenderness is over the medial femoral attachment of the ligament (which may help distinguish from true joint pathology).

If there is laxity of ligaments at neutral extension (0°) then always consider multiple ligament pathologies.

Imaging modalities

Radiography

Plain radiographs may demonstrate an avulsion fracture. In cases with a past history of MCL tear plain films may show ossification within the ligament, particularly proximally (Pellegrini–Stieda lesion).

Magnetic resonance imaging (MRI)

Findings include
- Full-thickness tears are seen as ligament discontinuity. Fig. 2.9 shows a full thickness disruption of the MCL (arrows).
- Minor low-grade strains and partial tears of the MCL will be seen as high signal on T2 imaging in and around the ligament.
- Bone bruising of the lateral aspect of the tibia and femur may be seen as a result of impaction sustained with valgus stress.

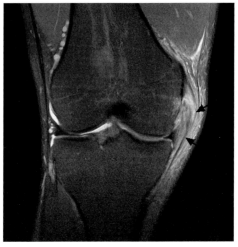

Fig. 2.9 Coronal MRI showing a full thickness MCL tear (arrows).

Lateral collateral ligament

Clinical features

Sporting injuries are probably the commonest cause for lateral collateral ligament (LCL) damage, especially with forced varus stress, although these are less common than MCL injuries. They are usually found in combination with other ligamentous injuries.

On examination, varus stress is painful and demonstrates laxity.

Imaging modalities

Radiography

- The lateral collateral ligament runs between the fibular head and lateral aspect of the lateral femoral condyle. There may be an avulsion fracture from the site of ligament insertion. Fig. 2.10a shows an avulsion of the LCL at its origin and the small avulsed fragment of bone is demonstrated adjacent to the lateral femoral condyle (arrow). Occasionally a small accessory ossicle (cymella) is seen associated with the popliteus tendon in a similar location and it is important to distinguish the two.

Magnetic resonance imaging (MRI)

Findings include:

- Fluid and haemorrhage will be seen around the torn ligament.
- In cases of a full-thickness tear ligament discontinuity will be seen. Fig. 2.10b shows a coronal MRI from the same case as Fig. 2.10a. The avulsed fragment of bone (arrowhead) is seen and the LCL itself (arrow) is shown extending between the avulsed fragment and the fibular head (F).
- Bone bruising of the medial aspect of the tibia and femur may be seen as a result of impaction sustained with valgus stress.
- A careful review of the cruciate ligaments and other structures of the posterolateral corner including the biceps and popliteus tendons is required as these structures are often injured with the LCL.

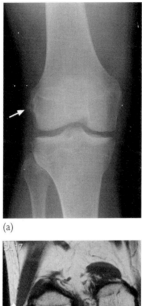

(a)

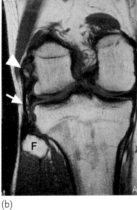

(b)

Fig. 2.10 (a) and (b) Avulsion of the LCL at its origin. There is a small avulsed fragment of bone demonstrated adjacent to the lateral femoral condyle on the AP radiograph (arrow). This is seen on the MRI (arrowhead) along with the avulsed ligament (arrow). F = fibula.

Patellar tendon (chronic injuries)

Clinical features

This is usually an overuse injury and presents often with pain most frequently localized to the inferior pole of the patella. Symptoms are worse with flexed weight-bearing activities such as walking up and down stairs.

On examination there may be pain on resisted extension of the knee, and tenderness on direct palpation (usually over the inferior pole).

Imaging modalities

Radiography

Plain radiographs may demonstrate:
- Thickening of the soft tissue stripe representing the patellar tendon
- Bone irregularity at the patellar tendon origin

Magnetic resonance imaging (MRI)

The characteristic features on MRI of tendinopathy (chronic tendon injury) are the same wherever they are seen in the body. The appearances are:
- Thickening of the tendon
- Abnormal increased signal on all sequences from within the tendon. Normal tendons show uniform low signal on all sequences. Fig. 2.11 shows abnormal increased signal in the thickened proximal patellar tendon (arrow) in a patient with proximal patella tendinopathy.

▶ It is important to see the increased signal on all sequences as increased signal may be seen in tendons on short TE (T1 and proton density) sequences as a result of artefact due to tendon position (known as magic angle effect).
- There may be inflammatory change in the adjacent tissues. In the case of patellar tendinopathy these are most often seen in the adjacent prepatellar fat pad (Hoffa's fat pad) and bursae. In Fig. 2.11 high signal oedema is seen adjacent to the patellar tendon in the fat pad (arrowhead)

Other imaging modalities

Patellar tendinopathy is also well seen on ultrasound as thickening of the tendon and low reflective change. Neovascularization may also be seen with Doppler imaging. In many centres this is the imaging modality of choice.

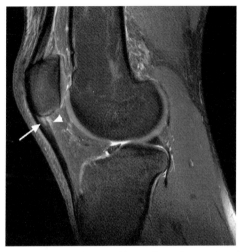

Fig. 2.11 Proximal patellar tendinopathy. There is abnormal increased signal in the thickened proximal patellar tendon (arrow). Note associated oedema in Hoffa's fat pad (arrowhead).

Patellar tendon (acute injuries)

Clinical features

Post-traumatic injury is the commonest cause of acute patellar tendon injuries. These present as full or partial ruptures with pain, swelling and marked loss of quadriceps function. Such tears usually occur in patients whose tendon is already weakened by chronic patellar tendinopathy.

On examination there may be swelling anterior to the knee, but a concavity in the region of the tendon may be present. Patella will migrate superiorly when there is a complete rupture.

Imaging modalities

Radiography

With complete tendon rupture plain radiographs may demonstrate elevation of the patella due to retraction of the quadriceps muscles. Fig. 2.12a shows a patient with a ruptured patella tendon and abnormally elevated patella (arrow).

Occasionally avulsion of the patellar tendon may be seen. This is usually seen in children (patellar sleeve avulsion fracture) where often only a small bone avulsion is observed but there is still a significant fracture as the patella inserts predominantly into non-ossified cartilage in the immature skeleton.

Magnetic resonance imaging (MRI)

MRI readily demonstrates discontinuity of the patellar tendon seen in acute patellar tendon rupture. Partial thickness tears are seen as fluid-illed fissures within the tendon. In both full and partial thickness tears there is usually evidence of background patellar tendinopathy.

Other imaging modalities

The features of patellar tendon tears are equally well demonstrated on ultrasound and in many centres this is the imaging modality of choice. Fig. 2.12b shows a longitudinal ultrasound of the same patient as Fig. 2.12a. The patella (PAT) is abnormally elevated exposing the anterior femur (Fem). The patellar tendon (arrowheads) is seen attaching to the tibia (Tib) however it is separated from the patellar by a gap (double-ended arrow). This is the site of the tear.

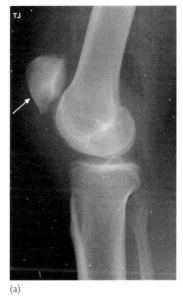

(a)

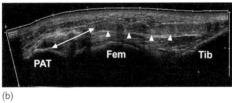

(b)

Fig. 2.12 (a) and (b) Lateral radiograph in patient with ruptured patella tendon. The patella (arrow) is abnormally elevated. The ultrasound from the same patient confirms a gap (double arrow) between the patellar tendon (arrowheads) and the patella (PAT). Fem = femur, Tib = tibia.

Quadriceps tendon

Clinical features

Trauma related to weight-bearing in flexion is the commonest cause of acute quadriceps tendon injuries. These may present with a sensation of something tearing or snapping in the suprapatella region of the leg. There is significant loss of quadriceps function.

On examination there may be swelling superior to the knee with some bruising. Look for focal tenderness and a concavity superior to the patella.

Imaging modalities

Radiography

Plain radiographs may demonstrate:
- Bone irregularity at the upper pole of the patella in chronic tendon disease
- Inferior displacement of the patellar and a joint effusion in cases of acute quadriceps tendon rupture

Magnetic resonance imaging (MRI)

In the case of acute tendon rupture MRI demonstrates:
- Discontinuity of the tendon
- A joint effusion

In chronic quadriceps tendinopathy MRI demonstrates:
- Thickening of the tendon
- Abnormal increased signal on all sequences from within the tendon.

Other imaging modalities

As with the patellar tendon these changes are also well shown on ultra-sound and in many centres this is the imaging modality of choice.

Bursae around the knee

Clinical features

Anatomically the bursae over the anterior knee are variable but typically comprise a pre patella bursa and superficial and deep infra-patellar bursae. Although pre-patellar bursitis is seen, the most common bursitis involves the superficial infra-patellar bursa which may become inflamed with chronic kneeling resulting in a large tender swelling below the patella.

Pes anserine bursitis usually presents as focal medial knee pain, often posteromedial in location, usually with gradual onset. It tends to present in people with abnormal biomechanical loading of the medial side of knee, e.g. people who walk with functional valgus gait.

▶Pes anserine bursitis may be confused with true medial joint pain, although it lies in an extra-articular position.

Imaging modalities

Radiography

Plain radiographs may demonstrate:
• Soft tissue swelling

Magnetic resonance imaging (MRI)

MRI demonstrates:
• A bursal effusion (IN the normal situation only a trace of fluid is seen)
• Synovial thickening in the bursa
• Edema in the adjacent soft tissues

All these features are show increased signal on T2 imaging.

Other imaging modalities

Bursitis is also well seen on ultrasound and is the imaging modality of choice in most centres. Fig. 2.13 shows a case of superficial infra-patellar bursitis. The bursa (arrowheads) overlies the inferior pole of the patella (Pat) and the patellar tendon (Ten). It is seen to contain anechoic fluid which appears black. The bursa is surrounded by subcutaneous fat and folds of fat extend into the bursa (f).

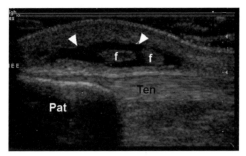

Fig. 2.13 Superficial infrapatella bursitis. The fluid filled bursa (arrowheads) overlies the patella (Pat) and patellar tendon (Ten). Folds of fat extend into the bursa (f).

Baker's cyst

Clinical features

A Baker's (popliteal) cyst arises as fluid fills a synovial lined outpouching of the posteromedial knee. A Baker's cyst may be a reflection of intra-articular knee pathology, usually osteoarthritis. However, they are not infrequently seen in young adults or even children without significant knee pathology. This cyst may or may not be symptomatic, and sometimes this relates to the size of the cyst.

Sometimes these cysts present on rupture with a story of acute pain and a sensation of fluid or swelling in the back of the calf. Pain may also arise as a result of chronic leakage of synovial fluid into the surrounding soft tissues.

Because the cyst communicates with the knee joint loose bodies may pass from the joint to the cyst.

On examination, there is a smooth, often non-tender, swelling in the concavity of the popliteal fossa. After rupture the swelling may not be present but there may be tenderness along the track of released fluid and sometimes some bruising.

▶ The major differential diagnosis is of deep venous thrombosis, especially in the case of ruptured cyst.

Imaging modalities

Radiography

Plain radiographs may demonstrate:
• Soft tissue swelling in the popliteal fossa
• Loose ossific bodies in the cyst
• Associated OA change within the knee joint

Magnetic resonance imaging (MRI)

MRI will demonstrate:
• The fluid-filled cyst (high signal on T2 imaging) in the posteromedial popliteal fossa. It characteristically arises from between the medial head of gastrocnemius and the semimembranosus tendons and as such can be reliably distinguished from other inflamed bursae in the popliteal fossa or other soft tissue masses.

The knee should be carefully examined for associated abnormalities such as meniscal tears and OA change.

If the cyst has leaked or ruptured:
• Pockets of fluid will be seen in the popliteal fossa and calf usually tracking superficial to the deep fascia of the gastrocnemius
• The residual cyst may also be seen

Other imaging modalities

Popliteal cysts are well seen on ultrasound with a characteristic appearance as they arise between the semimembranosus and medial gastrocnemius. Ultrasound is the imaging modality of choice and reliably demonstrates cyst rupture or leakage. Fig. 2.14a shows a Bakers cyst (*) arising from the back of the knee joint via a thin tract (arrow) which wraps around the medial aspect of the medial head of gastrocnemius (G). The configuration has been likened to a speech bubble and is characteristic of a Baker's cyst. Fig. 2.14b shows a different patient with a thick-walled Baker's cyst (black arrowheads) containing a large osteochondral loose body (arrow). This has a calcified centre which can be seen to cast a sonographic shadow behind the body (white arrowhead).

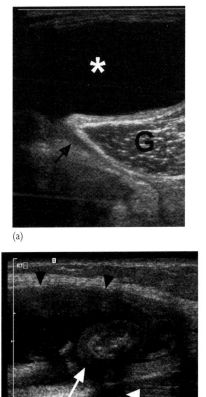

(a)

(b)

Fig. 2.14 (a) Ultrasound showing a Bakers cyst (*) arising from the back of the knee joint via a thin tract (arrow) which wraps around the medial aspect of the medial head of gastrocnemius (G). (b) is from a different patient with a thick-walled Baker's cyst (black arrowheads) containing a large osteochondral loose body (arrow). This has a calcified centre which can be seen to cast a sonographic shadow behind the body (white arrowhead).

Synovial masses

Clinical features

Besides generalized synovitis as a result of inflammatory or mechanical arthritis several specific conditions result in synovial hypertrophy. Imaging can have an important role in distinguishing these.

Synovial (osteo)chondromatosis

This condition results from benign synovial hypertrophy and metaplasia. The hypertrophied synovium forms cartilage nodules which may shed off into the joint becoming loose bodies. The bodies may ossify at which point the condition is usually know as synovial osteochondromatosis. Although any joint may be affected the knee is most one of the most frequently involved. The same condition can occur in synovial lined bursae.

Radiography

Plain radiographs may demonstrate:

- Multiple ossific bodies representing the ossified cartilage nodules. Fig. 2.15 shows an example (arrow points to multiple ossific bodies in the anterior knee)
- Rarely bone erosion from the synovial hypertrophy

Magnetic resonance imaging (MRI)

May demonstrate:

- A synovial mass
- Multiple bodies which may be loose or attached to the synovium. These will show low signal on all sequences if they are ossified completely, but their signal will depend on the amount of cartilage to bone in any nodule.

Pigmented villonodular synovitis (PVNS)

This is a benign condition resulting from synovial hypertrophy. It can occur in any synovial-ined structure including joints, tendon sheaths and bursae. The knee is the most common joint to be affected and the disease presents as a monoarthritis with insidious onset. Characteristically the synovial mass contains haemosiderin which gives it a pigmented appearance at histology and characteristic appearances on MRI.

Radiography

Plain radiographs may demonstrate:

- A joint effusion
- Soft-tissue swelling which is characteristically relatively dense due to the haemosiderin
- Rarely bone erosion from the synovial hypertrophy

Magnetic resonance imaging (MRI)

- A synovial mass which may be generalized or focal. The synovium may show typical signal characteristics of intermediate to relatively low signal on both T1- and T2-weighted imaging due to the haemosiderin. Synovial masses generally show high T2 signal. Fig. 2.16 shows an axial T2W image through the suprapatellar pouch of a knee, The suprapatellar pouch is filled by a mass showing intermediate to low signal (arrows). F, femur.

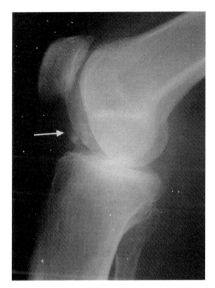

Fig. 2.15 Synovial osteochondromatosis seen as multiple ossific bodies (arrow) on this lateral knee radiograph.

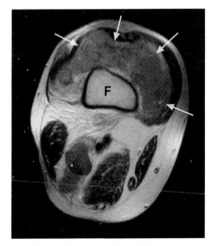

Fig. 2.16 Pigmented villonodular synovitis. Axial MRI shows the suprapatellar pouch is filled by a mass showing intermediate to low signal on this T2 weighted image (arrows). This is characteristic for PVNS. F = femur.

Fractures

Clinical features

Fractures around the knee include fractures of:

- The patella—usually the result of a direct blow.
- The femoral condyles—as a result of valgus or varus stress during severe axial loading.
- The tibial plateaus—these fractures are relatively common but can be difficult to diagnose. Minimal trauma may be involved in elderly patients especially if there is osteoporosis.

Imaging modalities

Radiography

While the fracture may be clearly visible these fractures, particularly those involving the tibial plateaus, can be subtle. The presence of a lipohaemarthrosis is an important sign indicating an intra-articular fracture.

- Lipohaemarthrosis results from the leakage of fat (from the bone marrow) and blood into the joint
- Fat floats on the joint fluid forming a fat–fluid level normally seen in the suprapatellar pouch in the supine position

Fig. 2.17 shows a lateral knee film obtained with the patient supine. The straight line representing the fat–fluid layer in the suprapatellar pouch is clearly seen (arrowheads).

For some fractures, particularly those involving the tibial plateau, plain films will fail to demonstrate the fracture, or fail to give a good indication of the complex 3D fracture configuration. In this situation CT is invaluable. It is particularly important for the surgeon to establish the degree of depression of the tibial plateau. Plain films underestimate this compared with CT.

Stress and insufficiency fractures

The knee is vulnerable to this type of fracture which may cause severe pain but be invisible on conventional radiographs. Stress fractures occur as a result of abnormal or repetitive force and may be encountered in athletes involved in running. The tibial plateau is a typical site. Insufficiency fractures result from the application of normal forces through abnormal bone. Osteoporosis is the most common bone abnormality associated with these fractures which typically occur in the subchondral bone of the femoral condyles or tibial plateaus.

Radiography

Plain films may show a sclerotic line representing the compressed and fractured trabeculae. However the findings are often very subtle and the fracture may be invisible.

Magnetic resonance imaging (MRI)

Fig. 2.18 shows (a) T1 and (b)T2 fat-suppressed coronal images through the knee of a keen amateur runner. MRI is extremely helpful typically showing a low signal line representing the fracture line (black arrow). The surrounding area shows marrow edema seen as high signal on fat-suppressed T2W imaging and intermediate to low signal on T1W imaging.

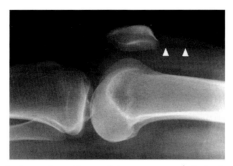

Fig. 2.17 Lipohaemarthrosis. The straight line representing the fat-fluid layer in the suprapatellar pouch is clearly seen (arrowheads).

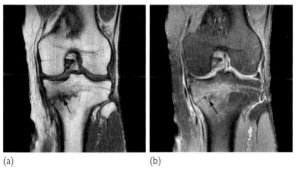

(a)   (b)

Fig. 2.18 (a) T1 and (b) T2 fat-suppressed coronal images through the knee of a keen amateur runner. A low signal line representing a fracture line (black arrow) is seen in the medial tibia. The surrounding area shows marrow edema seen as high signal on fat suppressed T2W imaging and intermediate to low signal on T1W imaging.

Investigating hip region problems

Anatomy

Bone and joint

The bony structures of the hip region are the innominate bone and the proximal femur. The innominate bone is formed from three individual bones: the ilium, the ischium, and the pubis. In adults these bones are fused together at the acetabulum but in children, prior to skeletal maturity, a Y-shaped cartilage, called the triradiate cartilage, separates them. The ischium and pubic bone also fuse together inferiorly where the inferior pubic ramus meets the ramus of the ischium. The left and right hip bones articulate with each other anteriorly at the pubic symphysis. Posteriorly, each hip bone articulates with the sacrum via the sacroiliac joints.

The hip joint is a synovial ball and socket joint where articulation occurs between the partially spherical femoral head and the concave acetabulum of the innominate bone. The acetabular socket is deepened by a rim of fibrocartilage called the labrum. This surrounds almost the entire rim but is deficient inferiorly at the site of a small acetabular notch. The articular surface of the acetabulum is horseshoe-shaped and covered by hyaline cartilage. Centrally, the acetabulum is non-articular and called the acetabular fossa. It contains a small fat pad.

The upper end of the femur consists of a head, neck, and two bony prominences, the trochanters. The head is about two-thirds of a sphere covered by hyaline cartilage but has a small pit in the centre called the fovea capitis. Within the hip joint, a thin ligament called the ligamentum teres inserts into the fovea capitis and to the margins of the acetabular notch. This ligament provides a small amount of the blood supply to the femoral head.

The femoral neck passes inferiorly, laterally, and posteriorly from the head to the shaft. At the oblique junction of the neck and the shaft, the greater trochanter lies laterally and superiorly while the lesser trochanter lies medially and inferiorly. The trochanters form the sites of attachment of important muscles/tendons.

The hip joint capsule attaches to the periphery of the acetabular labrum medially and laterally attaches to a line joining the femoral trochanters. The capsule is lined by synovium which also covers the ligamentum teres and the acetabular fossa fat pad. The capsule is thickened and strengthened by pubofemoral, ischiofemoral and iliofemoral ligaments, the latter being Y-shaped and strongest. A transverse acetabular ligament connects the inferior margins of the labrum across the acetabular notch, converting it into a tunnel through which blood vessels and nerves enter the joint. A small anterior opening in the joint capsule is frequently found between the pubofemoral and iliofemoral ligaments. A pouch of synovium protrudes through the opening and forms the iliopsoas bursa.

In addition to the small blood supply via the ligamentum teres, the proximal femur receives a much greater supply from vessels passing proximally through the capsule along the femoral neck. These vessels may be disrupted by intracapsular fractures of the neck of the femur.

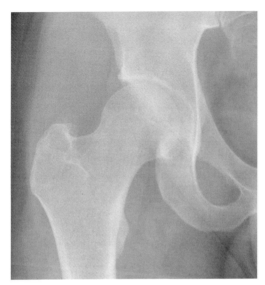

Fig. 3.1 AP view of the right hip joint.

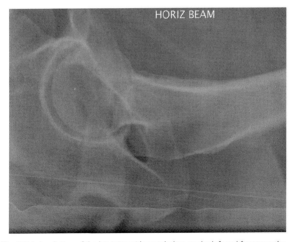

Fig. 3.2 Lateral view of the hip joint with acetabulum to the left and femur on the right side of the image.

Joint movements and soft tissue structures

As it is a ball and socket joint the hip has a wide range of movements, although less than that possible at the glenohumeral joint of the shoulder. The lesser movement range of the hip brings with it greater stability.

Flexion is mainly performed by iliopsoas (IP, inserting on the lesser trochanter), rectus femoris (RF, originating (1) at the anterior inferior iliac spine and (2) superior to the acetabulum, and sartorius (SA, originating at the anterior superior iliac spine).

Extension is mainly performed by gluteus maximus (GMAX, originating on the outer surface of the ilium behind posterior gluteal line, posterior surfaces of sacrum, coccyx and sacrotuberous ligament and inserting onto iliotibial band (ITB) and posterior femoral shaft) and the hamstring muscles (originating on the ischial tuberosity).

Abduction is mainly performed by gluteus medius and minimus (GMM), originating on the posterior ilium and inserting onto the greater trochanter.

Adduction is mainly performed by adductor longus, brevis and the adductor fibres of adductor magnus (originating from the pubis, inferior pubic ramus and ischial ramus and inserting on the linear aspera of the posterior surface of the femur).

External rotation is mainly performed by piriformis, obturator internus (OI), obturator externus, the gamelli and quadratus femoris (QF).

Internal rotation is mainly performed by gluteus medius/minimus anterior fibres and by tensor fasciae latae (TFL).

Imaging modalities

Radiography

- Useful to demonstrate normal alignment and position of bony structures
- Useful for initial investigation of arthritis and trauma
- Arthrography outlines joint capsule

Magnetic resonance imaging (MRI)

- Demonstrates soft tissue and bony structures
- More costly and may be difficult (claustrophobia) or contraindicated (some internal metal/devices) in some patients

Ultrasound (US)

- Less useful in the hip than, for example, the shoulder but still helpful for detection of joint effusions, especially in children
- Very helpful for dynamic conditions such as snapping hip
- Can guide injections/aspiration

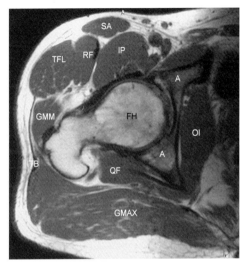

Fig. 3.3 Axial T1 MRI of right hip joint showing femoral head (FH) and acetabulum (A) in addition to some of the muscles listed above.

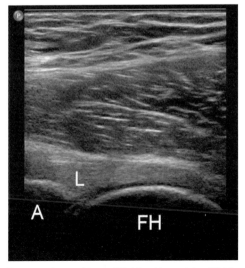

Fig. 3.4 Transverse ultrasound image of hip joint with acetabulum (A), labrum (L) and femoral head (FH) indicated.

Osteoarthritis of the hip

Clinical features

Osteoarthritis (OA) of the hip is uncommon before the age of 60 unless there is a predisposing structural abnormality (e.g. previous fracture, Perthes' disease or underlying inflammatory arthritis). Men and women are equally affected. Certain occupations such as farming seem to be a predisposing factor but obesity is not.

Pain is the most common presenting complaint. Often it is poorly localized and may be in the buttock, lateral aspect of the hip, groin or radiating to the knee. It is very rare for it to be felt below the knee. Pain is typically worse during or after activity but may disturb sleep. By the time patients seek attention for the pain there is usually restriction of hip movement and rotational movement is first affected. Apparent hip pain without restriction of movement should prompt the search for an alternative diagnosis, such as trochanteric bursitis, referral from the lumbar spine, or primary bone pathology, for example Paget's.

In general, there is good correlation between the clinical diagnosis of OA hip based on both history and examination and the radiological changes.

- hip OA affects about 5% of individuals over 60
- pain from the hip may radiate to the knee. Always examine the hip in a patient with knee pain
- the OA hip phenotype is fairly consistent—hip pain, sleep disturbance, restricted hip movement—particularly rotation—and loss of joint space on plain radiographs.

Imaging modalities

Radiography

Standard AP radiographs are the initial investigation of choice. Laterals should be included if a fracture is suspected. Radiological features of established OAs are:

- Irregular loss of joint space
- Osteophytes
- Subchondral cysts
- Subchondral sclerosis

Magnetic resonance imaging (MRI)

MRI will demonstrate cartilage loss and osteophytosis with greater sensitivity than radiography. It will also demonstrate subchondral bone abnormalities such as typical bone marrow lesions.

If plain radiographs are normal MRI may reveal cartilage loss and bone changes not apparent on standard radiographs or alternative explanations for symptoms such as psoas abscess, bone tumours.

MR arthrography is of value in assessment of femoro-acetabular impingement and labral pathology.

Other imaging modalities

Ultrasound is useful for identifying joint effusion and allowing aspiration and injection under guidance.

Hip arthrography with local anaesthetic injection is useful to distinguish between groin pain due to hip OA and that referred from lumbar spine degenerative disease.

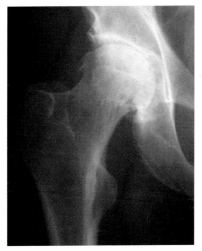

Fig. 3.5 A view of the right hip showing typical features of OA.

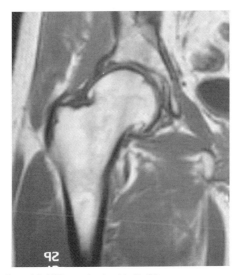

Fig. 3.6 Coronal T$_1$ MRI image showing right hip OA.

Inflammatory arthritis of the hip

Clinical features

The hip may be involved in all of the chronic inflammatory arthropathies (rheumatoid arthritis (RA), psoriatic arthritis, ankylosing spondylitis, enteropathic and reactive arthritis). The absence of rheumatoid factor tends to mark the 'non-RA' group. These are often collectively known as the 'seronegative' arthropathies and first presentation of an inflammatory arthritis in the hip suggests a seronegative disease. Sacroiliac and spinal involvement may also be present in this seronegative group.

Pain and restriction of movement are the cardinal clinical features. Morning immobility/stiffness is more prominent than in OA. In RA, hip involvement tends to occur late in the disease when peripheral joint involvement is well established. In the seronegative spondyloarthropathies, hip involvement, particularly in males, may occur early and in the absence of other peripheral joint disease.

Imaging modalities

Radiography

Plain radiographs are the initial investigation of choice. Full pelvis images allow assessment of the sacroiliac joints as well as demonstrating the hips. Typical changes within the hips include:

- periarticular osteopenia
- uniform loss of joint space
- erosions, though they may be difficult to detect in plain pelvic radiographs.

Osteophyte formation and subchondral sclerosis are typically minimal or absent indicating a lack of bone response to the insult.

Magnetic resonance imaging (MRI)

MRI with gadolinium enhancement is the investigation of choice when detection of synovitis is important. Unenhanced MRI cannot distinguish between joint fluid and vascular synovium.

Other imaging modalities

Ultrasonography may be useful for diagnosis of effusions or guiding therapeutic interventions.

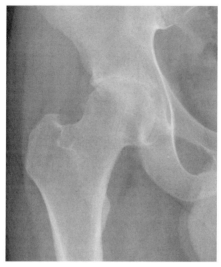

Fig. 3.7 Uniform loss of joint space, osteopenia and a muted bone response in this patient with rheumatoid arthritis.

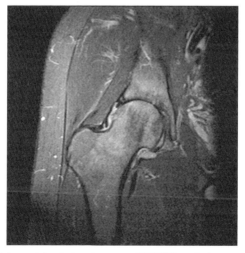

Fig. 3.8 A coronal short tau inversion recovery (STIR) MRI image in the same patient demonstrating bone marrow oedema, uniform cartilage loss and distension of the joint cavity with fluid signal material. Further MR imaging with contrast confirmed this to be synovitis not a joint effusion.

Infection around the hip

Clinical features

Septic arthritis is a medical emergency which needs to be investigated and managed as an inpatient. Involvement of the hip is more common in children under the age of one year where haematogenous spread occurs from adjacent osteomyelitis. The organism is most frequently *Staph. aureus.*

- In children, symptoms may be poorly localized and the presentation may be of an irritable, systemically unwell, febrile child. In adults the diagnosis should be suspected in any case of an acute or subacute monoarthritis of the hip.

- In adults, septic arthritis occurs most frequently in patients with an underling chronic arthritis, prosthetic joints, relevant comorbidities such as diabetes or alcoholism, the immunocompromised, or by direct inoculation in drug abusers. Again the causative agent is usually *Staph. aureus* but opportunistic infections may occur in the immunocompromised.

- Typically it is accompanied by systemic features and fever. However, with the increasing use of steroids, immunosuppression and biological therapies, clinical features may be markedly attenuated.

- Septic arthritis in prosthetic joints often presents considerable diagnostic challenge. Identifying the causative organism and its sensitivities is essential as antibiotic therapy may be required for several months or years.

- imaging is aimed towards aiding the aspiration of synovial fluid for culture (along with blood cultures).

Imaging modalities

Radiography

Plain radiographs are often normal or show periarticular osteopenia. They are useful as baseline images for charting subsequent changes.

Ultrasound (US)

Ultrasound is the investigation of choice coupled with joint aspiration.

Other imaging modalities

MRI is restricted in patients with prosthetic joints because of metal artefact due to the prosthesis. Radio-isotope bone scan or labelled white-cell scanning can be used but both have difficulty in distinguishing between inflammation, chronic infection, and loosening.

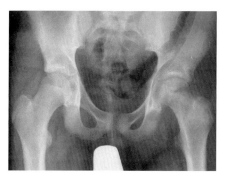

Fig. 3.9 AP view of a pelvis in a child with a left hip septic arthritis.

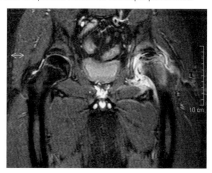

Fig. 3.10 Coronal short tau inversion recovery MRI image in the same patient as Fig. 3.9, showing a left hip joint effusion and bone marrow oedema in the femur and acetabulum.

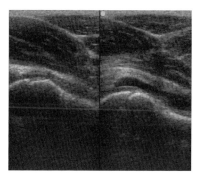

Fig. 3.11 Split ultrasound image showing normal hip on the left side and a hip joint effusion on the right.

Unusual hip pathology: osteoid osteoma

Clinical features

Osteoid osteomas are relatively rare, benign bone tumours of younger people which classically occur in the mid-diaphysis of a long bone, especially the tibia and femur. Symptoms are of pain, often more severe at night. Some osteoid osteomas are found close to or within joints, most frequently the hip, and here are often mis-diagnosed as arthritis. When intra-articular, the tumour incites considerable synovitis.

Imaging modalities

Osteoid osteoma within the hip joint can be difficult to diagnose on X-ray as the nidus is frequently difficult to identify without the sclerotic reaction normally seen surrounding osteoid osteoma of the shaft of a long bone. Subtle cortical thickening may be seen. Patients often undergo MRI where features suggesting synovitis are observed. Usually, bone marrow oedema is also seen, confined to the bone containing the osteoma, but the nidus may still be difficult to identify without a targeted CT study (see Fig. 3.12, osteoid osteoma nidus in left femoral neck (arrow)). Bone scan may be useful, demonstrating a 'double density' sign, but has a high radiation dose. Osteoid osteomas are commonly treated by CT guided percutaneous, minimally invasive techniques such as radiofrequency ablation.

Simple bone cyst

Clinical features

Simple bone cysts (SBC) are also termed unicameral bone cysts and are 'tumour-like' disturbances of bone growth, most common in the first two decades of life. SBC are most frequent in the proximal metaphyses of femur and humerus. Presentation is usually after fracture through the weakened bone.

Imaging modalities

On radiographs, SBC are slightly expansile lucent bone lesions lying centrally in the bone (see Fig. 3.13, SBC in left femoral neck) and frequently crossed by coarse 'pseudosepta'. After fracture, a piece of cortex may drop to the bottom of the cyst (fallen fragment sign). MRI shows uniform high T2 and low T1 signal without enhancement indicating fluid, although signal characteristics may change after fracture with fluid levels and high T1 signal due to haemorrhage.

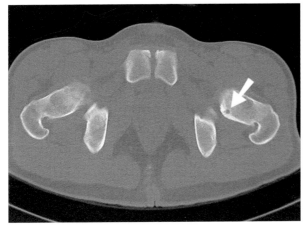

Fig. 3.12 Axial CT image showing a left femoral osteoid osteoma midus (arrow).

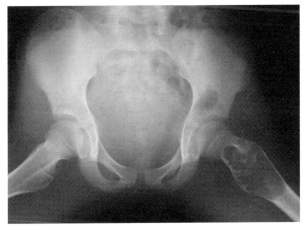

Fig. 3.13 'Frog leg' view of both hips in a child with a left femur SBC.

Malignant bone tumours

Clinical features

In adults, malignant lesions around the hip (Fig. 3.14) are most commonly metastatic deposits from primary tumours in breast, lung, prostate, and kidney, although a wide range of other malignancies can metastasize. Plasmacytoma, multiple myeloma, and lymphoma are also common causes of tumours of bone. Primary malignant tumours of bone include osteosarcoma, chondrosarcoma and Ewing sarcoma. These tumours are rare. Osteosarcoma (Fig. 3.15) and Ewing sarcoma are most common in young people, whilst chondrosarcoma is more typical in an older age group.

Imaging modalities

Radiography

The initial investigation and should be considered in patients of any age who are failing to respond to treatment for a suspected traumatic soft-tissue disorder or who complain of local pain and systemic symptoms such as weight loss. Most bone tumours around the hip appear as lucent bone lesions. The margins of the lesion give useful information about the aggressiveness of the tumour and the ability of the surrounding bone to respond to it. The presence of tumour matrix (calcification or ossification) can suggest chondrosarcoma or osteosarcoma.

Magnetic resonance imaging (MRI)

MRI is used for local staging. All patients with suspected primary malignant bone tumours should be referred to a specialist centre before biopsy to ensure subsequent treatment options are not compromised.

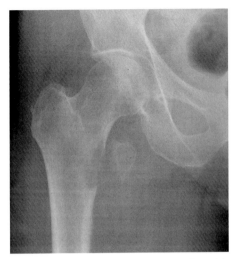

Fig. 3.14 AP radiograph demonstrating a lucent metastasis in the medial neck at the site of an avulsion of the lesser trochanter. This type of fracture is highly unusual in adults unless the underlying bone is abnormal.

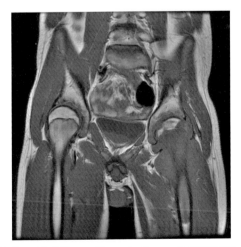

Fig. 3.15 Coronal T_1 MRI image of the proximal femora of a child showing replacement of normal bright (high) signal in the proximal left femoral shaft, neck and the outer (lateral) side of the epiphysis. A soft tissue mass also surrounds the neck. This patient has an osteosarcoma.

Acute hip fracture

Clinical features

Fracture of the proximal femur is a common injury in the elderly, linked to increasing frequency of osteoporosis and falls. Patients present unable to weight-bear with the affected leg shortened and externally rotated. Fractures of the proximal femur are classified according to the location of the fracture line with respect to the joint capsule.

Intracapsular fractures involve the femoral head and/or neck and may be:
- capital,
- subcapital,
- transcervical or
- basicervical.

Such fractures are associated with a relatively high incidence of complications such as avascular necrosis of the femoral head due to disruption of the capsular vessels which provide most of its blood supply. These injuries are therefore frequently treated by hemiarthroplasty.

Extracapsular fractures involve the trochanteric region and are classified as:
- intertrochanteric (see Figs 3.16 and 3.17) or
- subtrochanteric.

These injuries are typically treated with a dynamic hip screw (DHS). Blood supply to the trochanteric region is rich and osteonecrosis is unusual.

Fractures occurring after minimal/no trauma or at atypical sites, such as isolated fracture of the lesser trochanter, should prompt a search for an underlying bone lesion such as a metastatic deposit.

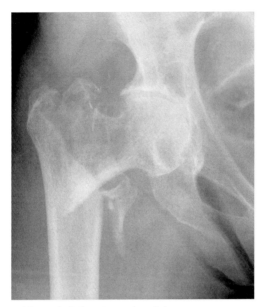

Fig. 3.16 AP view of right femur intertrochanteric fracture.

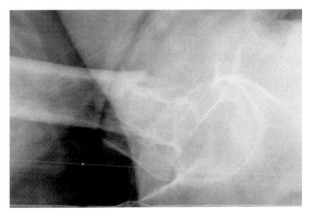

Fig. 3.17 Lateral view of right femur intertrochanteric fracture. Acetabulum is to the right.

Imaging modalities

Radiography

Radiographs are the investigation of choice and should consist of an AP projection and a lateral view. The diagnosis is commonly straightforward on the AP image when Shenton's line (following the medial cortex of femoral neck and inferior margin of superior pubic ramus) is disrupted.

Undisplaced femoral neck fractures can be difficult to identify and other imaging may be required.

Magnetic resonance imaging (MRI)

MRI is the gold standard imaging modality and also provides the most comprehensive assessment of other bone and soft-tissue structures which may be responsible for the pain (Fig. 3.19).

Other imaging modalities

Isotope bone scans will demonstrate linear uptake at the fracture site but can be confusing in the presence of extensive osteoarthritis.

CT frequently reveals a band of sclerosis at the site of a fracture and can often be obtained rapidly, useful in patients who may have difficulty remaining still due to discomfort (Fig. 3.18).

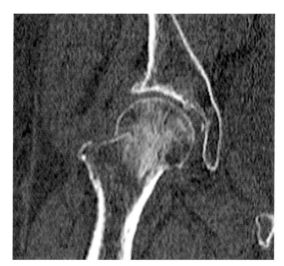

Fig. 3.18 Coronal CT reconstruction of the right femur neck in a patient with a subcapital fracture.

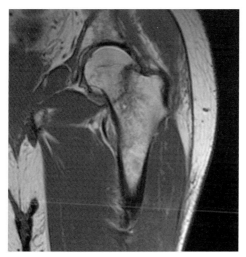

Fig. 3.19 Coronal T$_1$ MRI image of the left femur neck in a patient with a transcervical fracture.

Stress fractures around the hip

Clinical features

Bone requires stress for normal development and maintenance of trabecular density and organization. Stress may arise from weight-bearing or from muscular action. It is thought that microfractures occur and lead to remodelling and repair. Excessive force, such that damage exceeds the capacity for repair, leads to progressive fatigue and ultimate macroscopic fracture.

Stress injuries of bone comprise both injuries due to:

- abnormal stress applied to normal bone, e.g. excessive athletic activity in a runner leading to stress fracture of femoral neck
- normal stress applied to abnormal bone, e.g. fracture of the pubic rami and/or sacrum due to osteoporosis (such fractures are termed 'insufficiency fractures')

Stress fractures frequently present with insidious onset of pain and may be initially considered to indicate a soft-tissue injury or underlying sinister pathology. Having high clinical suspicion in at-risk patients is key to requesting appropriate imaging.

Imaging modalities

Radiography

Stress fractures may be visible on radiographs but are frequently normal initially. One of the earliest radiographic features is subtle loss of definition of an area of cortex (so-called 'grey cortex' sign) or of linear trabecular sclerosis in cancellous bone (Fig. 3.20). As the injury progresses, lucent fracture lines may appear.

Scintigraphy

Isotope bone scans (Fig. 3.21) readily demonstrate stress injuries of bone due to increased vascularity and osteoblast activity associated with them, but involve a high dose of ionizing radiation and provide little soft tissue information. They are useful when imaging of the whole body is required, such as when the differential diagnosis is of metastatic bone disease. Isolated uptake at a site of pain, without a linear orientation or suggestive history, frequently raises concerns about an underlying bone tumour.

Magnetic resonance imaging (MRI)

MRI represents the most useful imaging modality, with its great sensitivity to bone marrow oedema (Fig. 3.22), lack of ionizing radiation and ability to assess soft tissue structures.

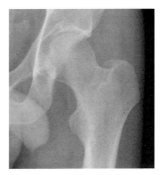

Fig. 3.20 AP view of left femur showing a subtle stress fracture of the inner side of the neck.

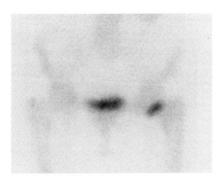

Fig. 3.21 Bone scan image of same patient as Fig. 3.21.

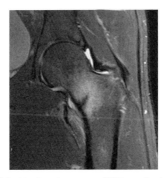

Fig. 3.22 Coronal short tau inversion recovery MRI image showing a left femoral neck stress fracture.

Avulsion fractures around the hip

Clinical features

Avulsion (apophyseal) fractures are injuries where forceful contraction of a ligament or tendon pull a fragment off the parent bone.

The majority of such injuries affect the maturing skeleton, occurring just before or after fusion of the apophysis, the secondary ossification centre, and the parent bone.

The muscle–tendon unit is stronger than the unfused or recently fused growth plate between the apophysis and remainder of the bone. A strong force thus results in a distraction injury of the apophysis rather than the injury of muscle which would be expected in a skeletally mature individual.

Avulsion fractures occur most often in activities requiring sudden bursts of speed such as sprinting, hurdling, or soccer. Sudden shooting pain is felt at the site of the apophysis. Local swelling may occur and the initial diagnosis may be of a soft-tissue injury. Healing occurs, frequently with exuberant callus. The imaging findings may be misinterpreted as a bone tumour.

The majority of avulsion fractures occur at the pelvic apophyses. Less frequently, avulsions of the iliopsoas insertion onto the lesser trochanter and the gluteal tendons onto the greater trochanter can be encountered.

When such injuries occur on older patients, an underlying bone tumour should be suspected.

Imaging modalities

Radiography

Avulsion fractures occur at anatomically predictable sites. X-rays therefore often show a linear bone fragment adjacent to a known site of tendon insertion. Fig. 3.23 shows avulsion of the origin of the rectus femoris at the anterior inferior iliac spine.

In chronic cases, exuberant callus is seen, and may again be misinterpreted as a bone tumour.

Magnetic resonance imaging (MRI)

When radiographs are negative, MRI is helpful, demonstrating bone marrow oedema and adjacent soft tissue oedema/haemorrhage at the site of the known apophysis. Fig. 3.24 shows partial separation of the right hamstring tendon origin from the ischial tuberosity (arrow) with reduced T1 signal in the tuberosity indicating bone marrow oedema.

Other imaging modalities

Bone scans show increased uptake but are non-specific.

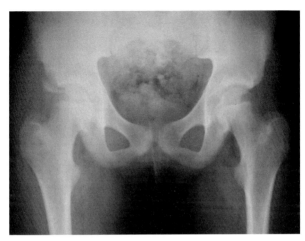

Fig. 3.23 AP view of a pelvis showing avulsion of the right rectus femoris origin at the anterior inferior iliac spine.

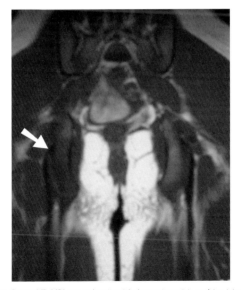

Fig. 3.24 Coronal T$_1$ MRI image showing right hamstring origin avulsion injury.

Avascular necrosis of the hip—adult

Clinical features

Avascular necrosis (AVN) of the femoral head is relatively common. The clinical challenge lies in the fact that symptoms, initially pain in the hip region, may occur before changes are apparent on plain radiographs.

Avascular necrosis results from interruption of the blood supply to the femoral head which mainly runs through the neck of the femur. This can occur for mechanical reasons such as a fractured neck of femur, or with increased blood viscosity as in the haemoglobinopathies.

It is well recognized in association with other diseases or therapies where the mechanisms are less well understood but appear to be associated with raised intraosseous pressure. These include Caisson's disease, alcoholism, pancreatitis, systemic lupus erythematosus, and corticosteroid therapy.

In the early stages pain is the main symptom. This may be sufficiently severe to prevent weight-bearing.

Imaging modalities

Radiography

Initial investigation is usually with plain radiographs. However examination and plain radiographs may be normal but an MRI will show marked changes in marrow appearance. Later, and this may take weeks or months to occur, structural changes occur in the femoral head (Fig. 3.25). The earliest are either a segment of increased bone density in the femoral head or a lucent thin crescentic line below the cortex (subcrescentic line). Later the ischaemic segment starts to collapse producing a 'sunken wedge' appearance but the joint space remains intact. Finally collapse of the femoral head and severe secondary OA occurs. By the time changes are present on plain radiographs it is extremely unlikely that any treatment other than hip arthroplasty will be effective. Some groups will undertake intraosseous decompression when only MRI changes are present.

Magnetic resonance imaging (MRI)

If there is a high index of suspicion, in the presence of a normal plain radiograph, MRI is the investigation of choice (Fig. 3.26).

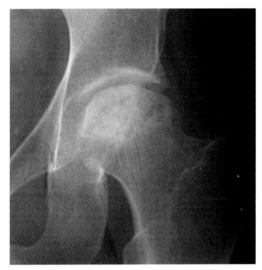

Fig. 3.25 AP view of left hip showing mixed sclerosis and lucency in established AVN.

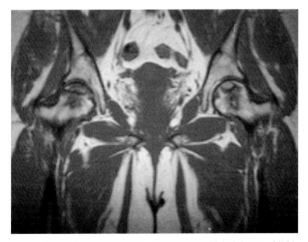

Fig. 3.26 Coronal T₁ MRI image of the pelvis showing established changes of AVN in both femoral heads.

Avascular necrosis of the hip—children

Clinical features

Osteonecrosis (avascular necrosis) of the proximal femoral epiphysis in children is also known as Legg–Calvé–Perthes disease, or more commonly, Perthes' disease.

- It is more frequent in boys than girls and typically occurs between the ages of 4 and 8 years.
- Occasionally (10% of cases), both hips are affected although not usually at the same time.
- Children present with a limp, pain, and restricted movement. The pain may be felt in the knee rather than hip area.
- The condition is self-limiting but the alteration in shape of the femoral head can predispose to secondary osteoarthritis as an adult. Involvement at an early age often has a better prognosis.

Imaging modalities

Radiography

At its earliest stage, Perthes disease is occult on radiographs, and MRI may be required. The earliest radiographic sign of Perthes' disease is local osteoporosis and periarticular soft tissue swelling but these are difficult features to detect reliably. Asymmetry of the size of the femoral epiphysis ossification centre may be seen. Most reliable, is the subcortical crescent sign (see Fig. 3.27) which is often better seen on the frog-lateral. Over time, sclerosis, flattening and fragmentation of the epiphysis occur (Fig. 3.28). Widening of the epiphysis and the femoral neck may be observed. Articular cartilage is maintained unless secondary osteoarthritis occurs and hence the joint space is not narrowed.

Magnetic resonance imaging (MRI)

In early disease with normal radiographs MRI can demonstrate changes in bone marrow signal characteristics in the proximal femoral epiphysis. There are significant difficulties in obtaining satisfactory MRI examinations in children in the typical Perthes' disease age range without general anaesthetic however and it is unusual for such examinations to be performed.

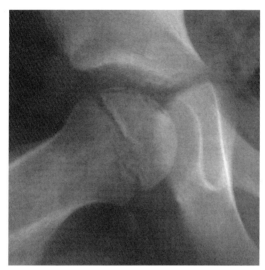

Fig. 3.27 'Frog leg' view of right hip in early Perthes disease showing subcortical crescent.

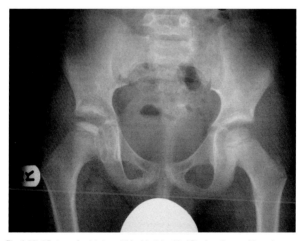

Fig. 3.28 AP view of pelvis in a child with right sided Perthes disease. Note the sclerotic flattened right femoral head.

Slipped capital femoral epiphysis

Clinical features

Slipped capital femoral epiphysis (SCFE) is a disorder where the epiphysis of the femoral head gradually moves posteriorly, medially, and inferiorly with respect to the neck. This occurs in adolescence due to weakness of the growth plate and is analogous to a chronic Salter–Harris type-1 fracture.

Boys are affected more frequently than girls, and SCFE is commoner in overweight children. Typical age range is 10–14 years. The left hip is more frequently affected in males, whilst in females, both sides are involved with a similar incidence. Although more commonly unilateral, bilateral involvement occurs in about a third of cases.

Children complain of pain in the hip, or sometimes knee, area. Clinical examination often detects limitation of movement and shortening of the leg.

Imaging modalities

Radiography

Early SCFE may be difficult to detect on a single AP view of the hip as the initial posterior displacement of the epiphysis causes only subtle loss of epiphysis height and blurring of the growth plate. Fig. 3.29 shows an early left SCFE. Frog-lateral views (Fig. 3.30) are of considerable value in detecting early cases by rotating the femur externally and allowing the slip to be more readily identified. It is useful to observe whether a line drawn along the lateral border of the femoral neck intersects the femoral head. Failure to do so indicates slip.

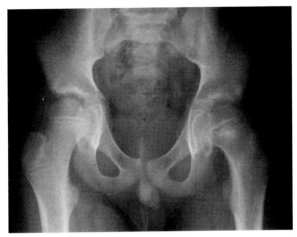

Fig. 3.29 AP radiograph of hips showing early left sided SCFE. Note the blurring of the left growth plate.

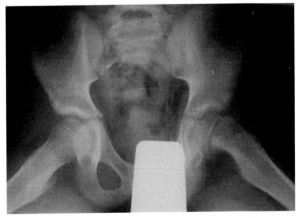

Fig. 3.30 'Frog leg' view in some patient as Fig. 3.29. The slip is now obvious.

Developmental dysplasia of the hip

Clinical features

This condition was previously termed 'congenital dislocation of the hip' (CDH) but developmental dysplasia (DDH) is preferred in order to acknowledge that many cases dislocate after birth.

DDH is much commoner in females than males (approximately 8:1) and has an incidence of 1.5 per 1000 births. The left hip is affected twice as often as the right hip and bilateral involvement occurs in 25% of cases. The condition is commoner in first-born children and there may be a family history.

Clinical diagnosis is established using the Ortolani and Barlow manoeuvres, however some children do not present until later, often when commencing to walk.

Imaging modalities

Radiography

The femoral head is not visible on radiographs taken at birth with ossification of the epiphysis occurring between 3 and 6 months of age. Radiographs can be used to assess the slope of the acetabular roof (acetabular index) and the relationship of the visible femoral neck to the acetabulum (Hilgenreiner line and Shenton–Menard line) but all such examinations result in exposure to ionizing radiation.

Ultrasound (US)

More recently, ultrasound has become the investigation of choice, allowing examination of babies at rest and with the hip under stress. Ultrasound is performed with the child lying on its side and the ultrasound probe orientated longitudinally to produce a coronal image of the side of the hip. This allows assessment of the slope of the acetabulum with respect to the surface of the ilium (alpha angle) and the cartilaginous acetabular coverage of the femoral head (beta angle). The former is most important and should be greater than 60° by the time the child is 3 months old. The effect of applied stress to the position of the femoral head can be assessed in real time using ultrasound and ready comparison with the opposite side is possible.

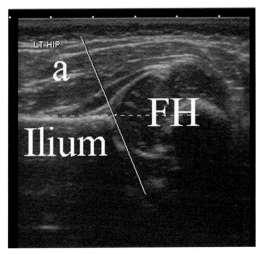

Fig. 3.31 Normal coronal ultrasound image of an infant hip. The alpha angle is marked (A). Note the position of the femoral head.

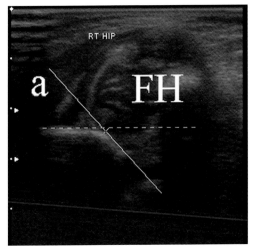

Fig. 3.32 Coronal ultrasound image of an infant with DDH. Note the reduced alpha angle (A) and the femoral head which lies much closer to the skin surface.

Transient osteoporosis of the hip

Clinical features

Transient regional osteoporosis (TOP) is a condition characterized by rapidly progressive osteoporosis of a localized area of periarticular bone, most commonly the femoral head, but which can affect other bones of the lower limb. A single area may be involved with symptoms typically lasting between 6 and 9 months before spontaneously regressing. There is no identifiable causative event and in some patients the disorder may recur in another area, when it is termed 'regional migratory osteoporosis'. Patients are most frequently pregnant women and middle-aged men, with the migratory form more common in the latter group.

The affected area is painful and local swelling may be detectable, although this is less easy to confirm in the hip.

Imaging modalities

Radiography

Radiographs may initially be normal until sufficient bone resorption takes place to allow the reduction in bone density to be appreciated, often by comparison with the normal contralateral side. Compare the lucent left femur with the normal right side in Fig. 3.33. As symptoms resolve, bone density increases on radiographs but follow-up imaging is not necessary to confirm this.

Scintigraphy

Bone scans are more sensitive in the early phase of the disorder but the appearances are not specific. The high radiation dose is a significant disadvantage of this modality and clearly contraindicated in pregnant women.

Magnetic resonance imaging (MRI)

MRI (Fig. 3.34) is also highly sensitive in detecting the bone marrow oedema, joint effusion and periosseous soft tissue oedema that characterizes the disorder and can differentiate between TOP and other potential concerns such as avascular necrosis or tumour. It is the investigation of choice in diagnosis, and where necessary, follow-up imaging.

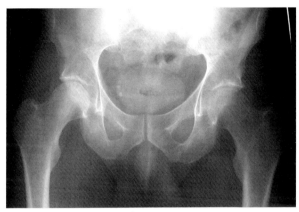

Fig. 3.33 AP radiograph in patient with left femur TOP. Note the reduced bone density.

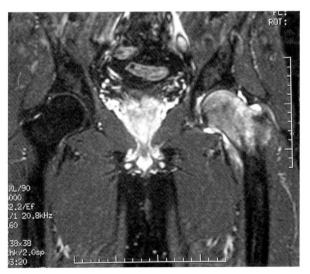

Fig. 3.34 Coronal short tau inversion recovery MND image in same patient as Fig. 3.33. Note the left hip joint effusion and bone marrow oedema in femoral head and neck.

Femoroacetabular impingement

Clinical features

Femoroacetabular impingement (FAI) is an important cause of early-onset osteoarthritis in an otherwise normal hip joint. FAI describes abnormal contact between the acetabulum and the femoral head–neck junction resulting in damage to the acetabular labrum and articular cartilage. Two distinct forms exist:

- Cam impingement, due to a non-spherical femoral head (typically due to a bump at the anterosuperior or lateral head–neck junction) which causes damage to the anterosuperior acetabular cartilage and labrum. Cam FAI typically affects young, athletic males.
- Pincer impingement, due to an excessively large acetabulum which 'over-covers' the femoral head leading to circumferential cartilage damage. Pincer FAI is typically found in middle-aged females.

Patients usually complain of a gradual onset of groin pain worsened by activity or sitting. On examination, symptoms may be reproduced by the impingement test where the hip is passively flexed, internally rotated and adducted.

Imaging modalities

Radiography

FAI may be diagnosed on radiographs prior to the development of classic osteoarthritis features.

- Cam impingement may be associated with a 'pistol grip' appearance of the proximal femur on an AP radiograph (see Fig. 3.35) due to the lateral head–neck bump.
- Pincer impingement is associated with protrusion acetabuli or acetabular retroversion.

Magnetic resonance imaging (MRI)

MRI arthrography allows more extensive evaluation of the joint, cartilage surfaces and aids detection of anterosuperior head-neck bumps (see Fig. 3.36) as well as detecting tears of the acetabular labrum which can be seen in association. Acetabular over-coverage can be assessed by directly observing the amount of femoral head surrounded by acetabulum in pincer impingement and the alpha angle, determined from the point at which the anterior surface of the femoral head ceases to be a smooth circle, can be calculated in cam impingement. In cam impingement the alpha angle is typically in excess of 50°.

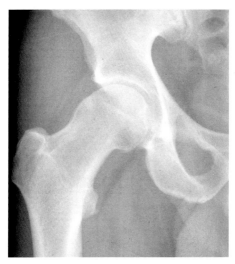

Fig. 3.35 AP view of right hip showing a 'pistol grip' femur.

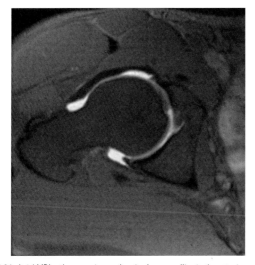

Fig. 3.36 Axial MRI arthrogram image showing bony swelling in the anterior surface of the femoral head/neck.

Labral tear

Clinical features

Tears of the acetabular labrum are a recognized cause of hip pain, often with a normal radiograph. Typical symptoms and signs are of persistent pain, clicking, restricted range of movement and locking. Pain is often felt in the anterior groin or thigh and worsened by flexion and internal rotation of the hip.

Injury can occur as a result of trauma, degeneration or due to underlying hip dysplasia. Traumatic labral tears often occur in the context of sporting activity and are related to twisting or pivoting injuries.

Imaging modalities

Radiography

The labrum is not visible on radiographs although X-rays may demonstrate a dysplastic hip joint or features of osteoarthritis.

Magnetic resonance imaging (MRI)

Conventional MRI has a low sensitivity in detecting tears of the labrum, particularly when large field of view (FOV) images covering the entire pelvis are used. Small FOV images covering only the hip itself have a slightly higher but still low sensitivity (25% sensitivity small FOV versus 8% sensitivity large FOV). MRI arthrography, performed with an intraarticular injection of dilute gadolinium contrast and using a small FOV, has been shown to be highly sensitive in detecting labral tears (92%) and is the investigation of choice. Most tears occur in the anterosuperior region of the labrum.

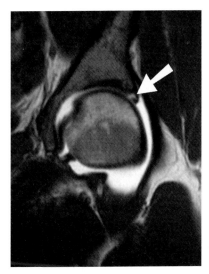

Fig. 3.37 Coronal T1 MRI arthrogram image demonstrating a tear of the anterosuperior labrum (arrow).

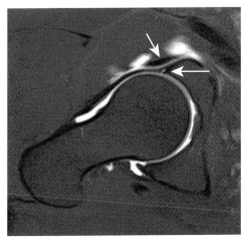

Fig. 3.38 Axial oblique fat-suppressed T1 MRI arthrogram image showing a tear of the anterior labrum (large arrow). Note the black psoas tendon immediately anterior to the labrum (small arrow) with injected contrast lying both medial and lateral to it. This contrast lies within an iliopsoas bursa, communicating directly with the hip joint in this patient.

Muscle injuries around the hip

Clinical features

Muscle injuries can be divided into:

- direct injuries where a laceration or blunt contusional force damages muscle tissue, for example compression of the vastus intermedius muscle against the femur during a rugby tackle
- indirect injuries where the force of muscle contraction overcomes the resistive forces within the locomotor chain linking the muscle via tendon to bone at each of its ends.

Indirect muscle injuries around the hip are common in young, athletic individuals although the location alters with increasing age. In adolescence, the weakest point of the locomotor chain is the secondary ossification centre where tendon attaches to bone. Hence juvenile sportsman more typically present with an avulsion fracture (📖 See Avulsion fractures around the hip, p.74), than a true muscle tear. After skeletal maturity, the musculotendinous (myotendinous) junction becomes the weakest segment of the chain and tears occur at this site. Muscles most at risk are those crossing two joints and with a higher proportion of 'fast twitch' fibres. Examples include rectus femoris in the quadriceps compartment, the hamstring muscles and sartorius.

Muscle tears are graded according to the severity of the injury and this provides useful prognostic information, especially in the professional athlete.

- Grade 1 injuries affect <5% of muscle volume on imaging and cause <5% loss of muscle function
- Grade 2 injuries affect >5% of muscle volume but do not cause complete rupture
- Grade 3 injuries are complete muscle tears with retraction of contracted tissue and result in complete loss of muscle function. The gap is filled with haemorrhage and debris.

Intramuscular haemorrhage is usually absorbed but occasionally peripheral calcification and subsequent ossification of the haematoma can occur, termed myositis ossificans.

Imaging modalities

Radiography

Radiographs have no useful role in the assessment of acute muscle injuries but may be helpful in subacute cases if myositis ossificans is suspected.

Ultrasound (US)

Ultrasound is useful in assessing large muscle injuries and in assessing the size and consistency of intramuscular haematoma. Small/subtle injuries may be more difficult to detect with ultrasound as symptoms may not be felt at the site of the injury. Ultrasound can assess muscle function dynamically.

Magnetic resonance imaging (MRI)

MRI readily detects small amounts of intramuscular haemorrhage/oedema and is the most sensitive modality for detecting acute injuries. It may require supplementation with ultrasound where large amounts of haematoma is present or where the dynamic assessment of muscle continuity is required.

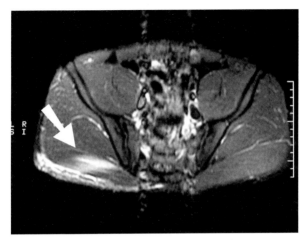

Fig. 3.39 Axial STIR MR image showing a grade 1 tear of gluteus maximus (arrow).

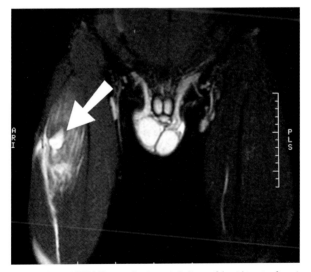

Fig. 3.40 Coronal STIR MR image showing a grade 2 tear of the right rectus femoris muscle within which an area of more focal haematoma can be identified (arrow).

Iliopsoas tendon/bursa

Clinical features

Hip pain may be caused by disorders of the iliopsoas tendon or arise from the iliopsoas bursa which communicates with the hip joint in 15% of the population.

Iliopsoas tear and tendinopathy may occur.

Iliopsoas bursitis can occur secondary to many hip joint disorders including osteoarthritis, rheumatoid arthritis, septic arthritis, gout, avascular necrosis or rare conditions such as synovial osteochondromatosis or pigmented villonodular synovitis.

It is typically treated by aspiration to exclude infection and thence antibiotics or steroids as required. This can readily be performed under ultrasound guidance. Treatment of the underlying hip disorder is necessary to prevent recurrence.

Snapping iliopsoas tendon is an interesting, dynamic condition typically affecting young female dancers, where the iliopsoas tendon and lower part of the iliacus muscle move anterior to the superior pubic ramus in a jerky rather than smooth fashion when the hip is moved from a flexed, externally rotated, abducted position back to a neutral position. Ultrasound is the only imaging modality which can assess this disorder.

Imaging modalities

Radiography

Radiographs can demonstrate the underlying hip joint abnormality but cannot visualize the bursa or tendon.

Magnetic resonance imaging (MRI)

MRI is useful for demonstration of the anatomy of the area and readily shows the iliopsoas tendon and muscle bellies, the tendon insertion on the lesser trochanter and the bursa when distended.

Ultrasound (US)

Ultrasound is useful for guidance of aspiration/injection and essential for the diagnosis of snapping iliopsoas tendon.

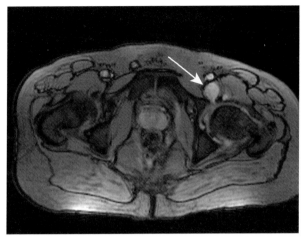

Fig. 3.41 Axial T2 gradient echo MR image showing a distended left iliopsoas bursa (arrow) which communicates with the hip joint via a slender neck located immediately medial to the iliopsoas tendon. A small additional component of the bursa lies lateral to the tendon.

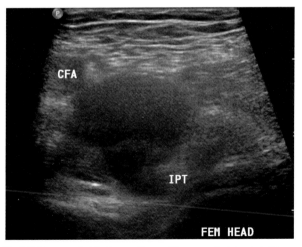

Fig. 3.42 Transverse (axial) ultrasound image of the same patient demonstrating the bursa and its relationship to the femoral head (fem head), iliopsoas tendon (IPT) and common femoral artery (CFA).

Trochanteric bursitis

Clinical features

Trochanteric bursitis or greater trochanteric pain syndrome (GTPS) is a common condition affecting middle aged adults.

The presentation is typically of unilateral hip pain, sometimes occurring after a period of increased activity. The pain localizes to the lateral side of the hip and disturbs the patient's sleep if they roll onto the affected side. On examination, the hip moves normally but there is well-localized tenderness to pressure over the greater trochanter.

The greater trochanter is the site of insertion of the gluteus medius and gluteus minimus tendons. Bursae are located between these tendons and the surface of the trochanter. Although the term 'trochanteric bursitis' is common in lay and medical use, most cases of GTPS are due to tendinopathy and tears of the tendons, analogous to rotator cuff disease in the shoulder. Distension of the bursae is rarely observed on imaging unless accompanied by tendinopathy and more commonly, tendon tear.

Very rarely a true infective bursitis may occur in the trochanteric bursa which can erode the greater trochanter and is frequently due to tuberculosis.

The diagnosis of GTPS is clinical with imaging rarely required.

Imaging modalities

Radiography

Plain radiographs are usually normal.

Magnetic resonance imaging (MRI)

Both MRI and ultrasound can demonstrate tendon thickening and tears with MRI also identifying oedema of tendon and surrounding soft tissue. MRI also more readily demonstrates atrophic changes in the gluteal muscle bellies occurring secondary to large tendon tears.

Ultrasound (US)

Ultrasound can also guide targeted injections.

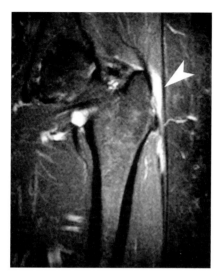

Fig. 3.43 Coronal STIR MR image of the left hip in a patient with GTPS. Note the bursal fluid collection (arrow) between the greater trochanter and the more superficial iliotibial tract.

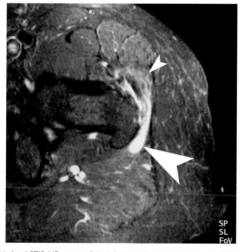

Fig. 3.44 Axial STIR MR image of the left hip in the same patient with GTPS. Note the bursal fluid collection (large arrow) and the tear and oedema of the gluteus medius muscle/tendon (small arrow).

Investigating shoulder region problems

Anatomy

The shoulder is the most complex joint in the body being a multi-axial spheroidal joint comprised of three articulations and two virtual ones:

- Glenohumeral joint
- Acromioclavicular joint
- Sternoclavicular joint
- Subacromial 'joint'
- Scapulothoracic 'joint'

The glenohumeral (GH) joint comprises the articulation between the humeral head and the glenoid of the scapula. As the articular surface of the glenoid is shallow a cartilage cuff surrounds the margins of the glenoid to increase its surface area. The synovial cavity is extensive with redundancy to allow for greater range of motion. Most of the movement of the shoulder occurs at this joint.

The fibrocartilagenous acromioclavicular (AC) joint occurs between the tip of the acromion and the lateral end of the clavicle. Its main purpose is to stabilize the shoulder.

The synovial sternoclavicular joint occurs between the medial end of the clavicle and the superolateral aspect of the sternum. It allows increased manoeuvrability of the shoulder, especially abduction.

The subacromial space, although not a true joint, lies between the under surface of the acromion and the superior aspect of the humeral head. It is crucial for the normal functioning of the shoulder, especially abduction.

The scapulothoracic 'articulation', again not a true joint, occurs between the under-surface of the scapula and the posterior aspect of the thoracic wall. Without this, abduction of the shoulder beyond 90° would not be possible.

The capsule of the joint itself is a synovial lined, fibrous structure which is loose and allows up to 3cm of separation of the bones. The normal intra-articular volume is between 20–50ml with thickenings of the capsule aiding support (glenohumeral ligaments). The coracoacromial, coracohumeral and transverse humeral ligaments also lend support.

The main stabilizing structure of the shoulder is the musculotendinous complex referred to as the rotator cuff. Parts of the tendons are fused with the shoulder capsule. The rotator cuff is involved with most movements of the shoulder joint and comprises:

- Supraspinatus
- Infraspinatus
- Subscapularis
- Teres minor
- +/– Long head of biceps

The supraspinatus muscle, arising from the supraspinatus fossa of the scapula and inserting into the greater tuberosity of the humerus, is the chief rotator cuff muscle and is responsible for the initiation of abduction.

The infraspinatus originates from the posterior aspect of the scapula inferior to its spine, inserts into the posterosuperior aspect of the greater tuberosity and is responsible for external rotation.

Teres minor originates along the axillary border of the scapula inserting into the posteroinferior aspect of the greater tuberosity (the muscle assists infraspinatus as an external rotator).

Subscapularis originates from the subscapular fossa and inserts into the lesser tuberosity of the humerus lateral to the glenoid labrum. It is separated from the rest of the rotator cuff by the bicipital groove. The principle action of this muscle is to internally rotate the adducted arm.

The long head of biceps arises from the superior aspect of the glenoid labrum and the short head arises from the coracoid process inserting into the radial tuberosity. Although not strictly a rotator cuff muscle it is intimately involved with the integrity of the cuff and is responsible for elbow flexion and forearm supination.

The subacromial bursa is the largest and most important bursa which lies between the deltoid muscle and joint capsule laterally and under the acromion and coraco–acromial ligament medially.

The shoulder is supplied by the suprascapular and axillary nerves.

Imaging modalities

Radiography

- Useful to demonstrate the normal alignment and positions of bony structures (Fig. 4.1).
- Arthrography will clearly outline the extent of the shoulder capsule (Fig. 4.2).

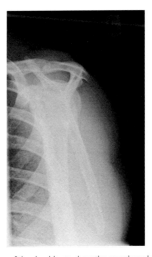

Fig. 4.1 Oblique view of the shoulder to show the scapula end on. This allows accurate determination of the humeral head in relation to the glenoid.

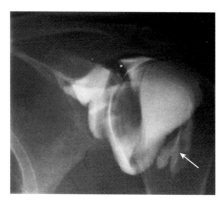

Fig. 4.2 Arthrogram of the left shoulder. Contrast medium has been injected into the joint. The extent of the capsule is demonstrated with fluid tracking down the bicipital tendon sheath(arrow). This is normal and results from the fact that the biceps tendon has an intra articular course proximally.

Ultrasound (US)
- Extremely useful to define the normal soft-tissue anatomy of the shoulder structures
- Particularly good for imaging the rotator cuff tendons and the subacromial bursa
- Limitation of being operator dependent

Magnetic resonance imaging (MRI) (Fig. 4.3, 4.4)
- Extremely useful modality for imaging the shoulder
- Demonstrates clearly almost all of the shoulder structures
- Limitations of cost, access and certain contraindications (e.g. claustrophobia, pacemaker)

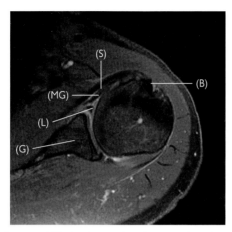

Fig. 4.3 Fat saturated (FS) T1 arthrogram of the glenohumeral joint showing the subscapularis(S), the biceps tendon(B), the middle glenohumeral ligament (MG), the glenoid(G) and the labrum(L).

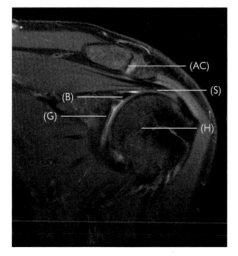

Fig. 4.4 Coronal oblique FS T1 MR arthrogram showing AC joint(AC), biceps origin(B), supraspinatus tendon(S), glenoid(G) and humeral head(H).

Glenohumeral arthritis

The glenohumeral joint is commonly involved in inflammatory arthritis (up to 90% in rheumatoid arthritis). Degenerative disease occurs with increasing age and secondary to inflammatory disease. Crystal disease may also involve the shoulder joint.

Clinical features

- Usually in those >40 years (degenerative disease in older age groups)
- Chronic deep-seated pain affecting the whole shoulder (often felt as if originating from the deltoid muscle)
- Aggravated by activity and relieved with rest (opposite is true with inflammatory disease)
- Pain may interfere with sleep
- Stiffness (greater than 30min duration if inflammatory)
- Swelling occurs with inflammatory and crystal disease
- Palpable or audible crepitus indicates grating of bony surfaces
- Globally reduced passive and active range of movement especially external rotation and abduction
- True glenohumeral movement only occurs up to 90° of abduction

A full assessment for a generalized inflammatory arthritis should be considered in anyone who complains of arthritic pain of the shoulder joint.

The cervical spine should always be assessed in cases of shoulder pain as radiation of pain from the neck is frequently felt in the shoulder region. Pain in the shoulder may also originate from the thorax (e.g. ischaemic cardiac disease) or abdomen (eg. cholecystitis).

Imaging modalities

Radiography (Fig. 4.5)

Typical findings include:

- narrowing of the joint space
- irregularity of the joint surfaces
- osteophyte development
- soft tissue swelling

No further radiological investigation is required if the clinical diagnosis is glenohumeral osteoarthritis unless the patient is being considered for surgery. It is then necessary to assess the whole shoulder 'unit'.

Ultrasound (US)

Ultrasound is frequently used to assess inflammatory arthritis and may show:

- Joint effusion
- Synovial thickening
- Increased vascularity (using colour-flow Doppler ultrasound)
- Ultrasound does not image the bone

Magnetic resonance imaging (MRI)

Similar to ultrasound, MRI can be a useful adjunct assessing inflammatory arthritis. Findings include:

- Joint effusion
- Synovial thickening
- Bony and cartilage changes can be apparent on MRI

See Fig. 4.5.

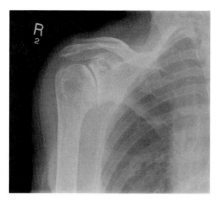

Fig. 4.5 Degenerative change of the right glenohumeral joint. Note the joint space narrowing, particularly inferiorly. Osteophytes are also seen at the inferior margin of the joint.

Acute dislocation

Anterior dislocation accounts for 98% of cases and follows forced abduction, external rotation, and extension of the shoulder. Posterior dislocation is rare and occurs following trauma, epilepsy or electric shock. Recurrent dislocations are common (up to 80%).

Clinical features

- Disorder predominantly of those in the teenage years to young adulthood
- Most frequent in females and those with hypermobility and/or ligamentous laxity
- The main complaint is of sudden onset excruciating pain in the shoulder region
- Deformity of the shoulder with a bulge anteriorly or posteriorly
- Anterior dislocations cause a 'square-shoulder' appearance with marked prominence of the acromion
- The arm is held in slight abduction and external rotation
- There is usually limitation of internal rotation and adduction
- Complete loss of movement of the shoulder may occur secondary to the anatomical derangement and pain
- There may be an associated rotator cuff tear especially in middle age
- Dislocation may lead to humeral head damage and increases the risk of future instability and arthritis

Following dislocation, the antero–inferior part of the capsule and labrum are often torn off the glenoid, occasionally with a bony fragment (Bankart lesion). A Hill–Sachs lesion is a compression fracture of the posterior surface of the humeral head following impaction against the anterior glenoid rim and may accompany a Bankart lesion.

Imaging modalities

Radiography (see Figs 4.6, 4.7 and 4.8)

- The head of the humerus is no longer located in the glenoid and may be displaced inferior, anterior or posterior to the glenoid fossa
- Two orthogonal views will be required if the dislocation is subtle or subluxation has occurred

Ultrasound (US)

- Does not have a role in the diagnosis either of acute dislocation, nor of the evaluation of the joint after dislocation

Magnetic resonance imaging (MRI) (see Fig. 4.8)

- MRI is not usually needed to diagnose shoulder dislocation
- Can be useful in determining the nature and degree of labral or glenoid damage that has occurred as a result of dislocation

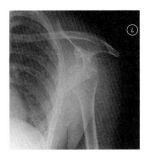

Fig. 4.6 Acute anterior dislocation of the right shoulder. The humeral head can be seen sitting anterior and inferior to the glenoid.

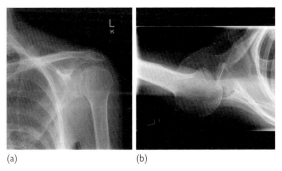

(a)   (b)

Fig. 4.7 (a) and (b) Locked posterior dislocation. The anatomical relation of the humeral head is difficult to determine on the frontal film, but the axial film shows that the posterior head is dislocated posteriorly, and is locked in that position by a 'divot' on the anterior aspect of the humeral head.

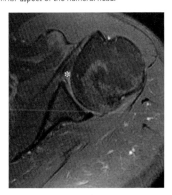

Fig. 4.8 MR showing anterior glenoid labral tear (*) following dislocation of the shoulder.

Anterior instability

Glenohumeral instability occurs when there is an inability to maintain the humeral head within the glenoid fossa. Subluxation or dislocation are common sequelae.

Clinical features

- Usually first presents in those <30 years
- Pain is episodic and occurs following certain movements such as throwing (invariably this occurs with the arm in the outstretched, i.e. abducted and externally rotated) or overhead position
- Clicks, if painful, may be a manifestation of instability
- Clunks are a feature of major instability
- 'Dead arm syndrome' of transient numbness, tingling and weakness of the arm or hand after throwing a ball with associated pain and subsequent dull ache is practically pathognomonic of shoulder subluxation
- There may be a history of weight training, swimming, and throwing sports
- Full active and passive range of movement is retained
- Impingement may be present (see 📖 p.126)
- With the patient relaxed the humeral head may be rocked backwards and forwards in the glenoid fossa

Apprehension test for anterior instability

With the patient lying supine on the couch, pain and anxiety may develop when the arm is abducted and externally rotated ('javelin' position). Applying anterior pressure to the upper humerus often relieves the discomfort and further external rotation may then be possible. When this stabilizing force is removed, symptoms return.

Repeated episodes of instability may lead to increased stress on the rotator cuff and other stabilizing structures giving rise to impingement and tendinopathy. Tendinosis is a frequent manifestation of underlying instability in the young athlete.

Imaging modalities

Radiography

- The shape of the bones is normal, and therefore no abnormality will be seen with uncomplicated instability.

Ultrasound (US)

- The appearances will be normal.

Magnetic resonance imaging (MRI)

- Although MR images the glenoid labrum well, the shape of this structure is highly variable and therefore MR it is not useful in this context.
- If there has been previous dislocation, MR will show evidence of bony or labral damage that has occurred as a result.

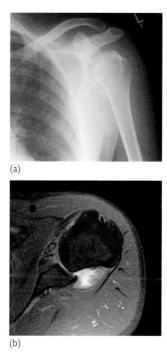

(a)

(b)

Fig. 4.9 (a) The shoulder has previously been dislocated, and is now in its normal position. However there is a fracture fragment inferior to the glenoid.
(b) Corresponding MR examination in this patient shows the bony Bankart lesion. The anterior portion of the glenoid is missing.

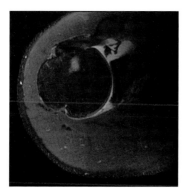

Fig. 4.10 MR arthrogram shows that the anterior labrum is torn and detached anteriorly.

Posterior instability

Posterior instability and dislocation are features of congenital laxity and multidirectional instability (see below).

Clinical features

Frequently missed, posterior dislocation may be identified by:
- a concavity below the acromion
- anterior deltoid flattening
- palpable humeral head posteriorly
- the arm held in adduction and/or internal rotation
- lack of active and passive external rotation

Posterior instability may be assessed by applying axial (downward) pressure to the flexed, adducted, and internally rotated arm (arm positioned across chest). The patient may then complain of pain or an impending feeling of joint dislocation.

Sequelae include fracture of the glenoid rim and proximal humerus (a reverse Hill–Sacks lesion).

Imaging modalities

Radiography
- If instability has lead to dislocation, then the abnormal position of the humeral head will be well seen on an axial view
- A frontal view may show the typical 'light bulb' appearance (see Fig. 4.11)

Ultrasound (US)
- Not useful in this context

Magnetic resonance imaging (MRI)
- Posterior dislocation may be associated with damage to the posterior aspect of the labrum (see Fig. 4.12).

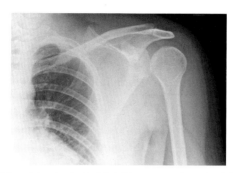

Fig. 4.11 Frontal view showing the 'light bulb' appearance of posterior dislocation.

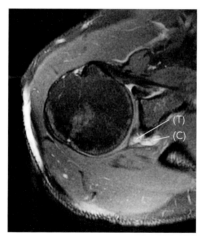

Fig. 4.12 Axial MR image of the shoulder showing tear of the posterior labrum(T). Fluid has forced through the tear to produce a power labral cyst(C).

Multidirectional instability

Multidirectional instability is usually seen in those with generalized ligamentous laxity/hypermobility. This leads particularly to a stretched, and thus redundant, inferior joint capsule. Minimal trauma causing the first dislocation may suggest pre-existing shoulder ligament laxity.

Clinical features

- Usually first presents in teenagers or young adults
- Symptoms are episodic
- Pain is felt in the anterior and/or posterior aspect of the glenohumeral joint, however this depends upon the main direction of instability
- Joint clicks are uncommon
- Weakness of the arm may be present in acute episodes
- A painful arc may be present
- Full active and passive movement is retained
- Impingement may be evident (see 📖 p.126)
- The shoulder will sublux inferiorly with traction on the arm (sulcus sign) in multidirectional instability and can be pushed both anteriorly and posteriorly with respect to the glenoid (drawer test)

Patients with multidirectional instability should be assessed for generalized ligamentous laxity. The true disorders of connective tissue (ie. Ehlers–Danlos syndrome, osteogenesis imperfecta and Marfan's syndrome) may all present with multidirectional instability.

Imaging modalities

Radiography (Fig. 4.13)

- As multidirectional instability normally results from laxity of soft tissues, no abnormality seen on plain film which images the bones

Ultrasound (US)

- Usually normal in uncomplicated multidirectional instability

Magnetic resonance imaging (MRI)

- Also normal in uncomplicated cases

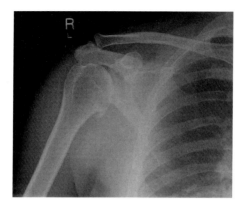

Fig. 4.13 Plain film shows an osteophyte on the inferior surface of the humeral head, with little in the way of degenerative change. This configuration suggests that there is excessive movement between the humerus and the glenoid, as a result of multidirectional instability.

Superior labral anterior–posterior (SLAP) lesions

The SLAP lesion is used to describe a tear of the superior labrum in the anterior–posterior direction. This type of injury is not uncommon and may occur following trauma in patients with underlying instability of the shoulder. A SLAP lesion may itself lead to instability.

Clinical features

- Usually in those <40 years
- Acute or chronic onset of deep seated poorly localised shoulder pain
- Weakness of the arm is not a feature
- There may be a history of subluxation, dislocation or repetitive microtrauma
- A fall on an outstretched hand may also be a precipitant
- Wasting is not present and a painful arc is uncommon
- Normal active and passive range of movement
- Impingement may or may not be present
- Signs of instability (📖 Anterior instability, p.106, Posterior instability, p.108)
- Internal rotation of the arm may precipitate catching, clunking or snapping of the shoulder

This is typically seen in throwers when excessive force is applied to the tendon of long head of biceps where it inserts into the superior labrum. The resulting instability may lead to disorders of the rotator cuff and long head of biceps.

Imaging modalities

Radiography

- The damage has occurred to the soft tissues, and therefore is not seen on plain film

Ultrasound (US)

- Intra-articular structures are not seen by ultrasound
- Other than secondary damage to the biceps tendon, the ultrasound will be normal.

Magnetic resonance imaging (MRI)

Very useful for determining patients who have a SLAP lesion:

- Linear high signal in the superior labrum
- This may extend into the insertion of the biceps (bicipital anchor)
- The tear may extend anteriorly or posteriorly
- A joint effusion is a common accompanying factor
- The underlying bony glenoid is normal

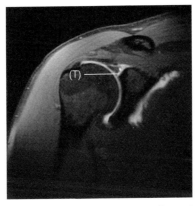

Fig. 4.14 Coronal oblique MR arthrogram shows a tear in the superior labrum(T).

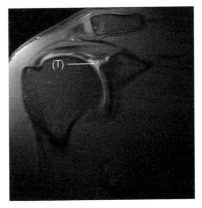

Fig. 4.15 Coronal oblique MR arthrogram shows tear and disruption of the anterior labrum anterosuperiorly(T).

Ageing of the rotator cuff

Disorders of the rotator cuff are very common and the majority occur in the absence of systemic disease. Partial interruption of the blood supply following injury may lead to incomplete healing and regeneration rendering the tissues more vulnerable with ageing. Cadaveric studies have shown a prevalence of up to 37/100 for partial thickness and 27/100 for full thickness tears (Fig. 4.16).

Clinical features

- Not all rotator cuff lesions are symptomatic
- The presence of imaging-detected pathology in the shoulder does not mean this is necessarily the source of pain in this region
- Careful history and examination are required to differentiate referred neck or acromioclavicular joint pain from true shoulder pain

Imaging modalities

Radiography

- Chronic damage to the rotator cuff is associated with cranial migration of the humeral head
- In the worse cases the humeral head can be seen abutting the under-surface of the acromion

Ultrasound (US)

- The supraspinatus tendon may be torn and retracted back under the clavicle to the extent that the tendon cannot be seen at all, resulting in the deltoid abutting the humeral head

Magnetic resonance imaging (MRI) (Fig. 4.17)

Usually superfluous, but if performed will show:
- Cranial migration of the humeral head
- Full thickness tear of the supraspinatus tendon
- Retraction of supraspinatus tendon by several centimetres
- Accompanying tears of the infraspinatus, subscapularis and long head of biceps (a common finding)
- Frequently a joint effusion is present with fluid having passed through the tear into the subacromial subdeltoid bursa

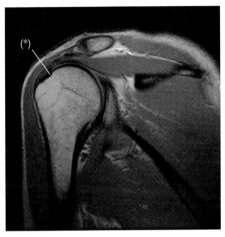

Fig. 4.16 MR coronal of the T2WI shows high signal within the supraspinatus tendon with diffuse tendinosis. This degree of tendinosis should be considered normal in this 75-year-old(*).

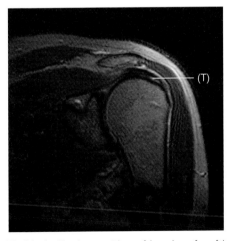

Fig. 4.17 MR of the shoulder shows partial tear of the under surface of the supraspinatus tendon(T).

Rotator cuff tears

The majority of shoulder pathology is secondary to rotator cuff damage which includes wear of the cuff (tendinosis) and tears. Supraspinatus is by far the most frequently affected musculotendinous unit followed by infraspinatus. Combined lesions are common and subscapularis and teres minor are rarely involved in isolation.

Tears of the rotator cuff may be classified as:
- Partial thickness (bursal and/or humeral side) refers to those where the tendon is torn or frayed but is intact overall
- Full thickness describes tears which have passed right through the tendon substance allowing one to 'see through' the tendon. Fibres may still be intact around this area of tear
- Complete refers to total disruption of the tendon where there are no intact fibres present and retraction has occurred
- Rupture of the cuff refers to a very large complete tear

Clinical features
- Usually occur in those >40 years
- Insidious or sudden onset of pain in the shoulder region
- Often aching in nature and poorly localized
- History of trauma may be present
- Night pain is prominent and the patient has difficulty sleeping on the affected side
- Work involving repetitive movements or heavy lifting may give rise to tears of insidious onset and this activity may exacerbate symptoms
- Muscle wasting around the shoulder may be evident
- A painful arc and weakness may be prominent
- Signs of impingement are pronounced, so this may present as subacromial impingement (📖 See p.126)
- There is restriction of movement of the shoulder (passive movement much greater than active)
- Total loss of active movement occurs with complete tears and rupture

A full range of movement may be retained in partial and full-thickness tears but may be limited by pain. Classically a painful arc is present between 60–120° of abduction, however in practice pain is often present throughout the movement.

Imaging modalities
Radiography
- Degenerative change of the AC joint is common
- There may be impingement changes in the greater tuberosity
- The soft tissue structures themselves are not seen

Ultrasound (US) (Fig. 4.18)
An excellent modality to assess the rotator cuff.
- The most commonly affected tendon (supraspinatus) is very well imaged
- With complete rupture and retraction of the supraspinatus tendon the deltoid abuts the humeral head as no interposing tendinous structure is present

- Full-thickness tear without retraction shows a concave anterior tendon border and the torn ends of the tendon may be visualized
- Partial thickness tears are seen as a focal discontinuity of the fibrillar pattern
- Altered signal within the tendon indicates tendinosis which commonly accompanies tears
- Other rotator cuff muscles and tendons are also seen on ultrasound but isolated tears of these structures are uncommon

Magnetic resonance imaging (MRI) (Figs. 4.19–23)

Excellent at determining partial and full-thickness rotator cuff tears. Features include:

- High signal within the supraspinatus tendon, particularly anteriorly towards the insertion on the fluid sensitive-sequence, indicates areas of tendon damage
- A partial tendon tear will show an area of high signal that fails to cross the full thickness of the tendon
- In a full-thickness tear, the high signal crosses the full thickness of the tendon
- The retracted end of the tendon will be seen in a complete tear and the amount of retraction can be quantified in centimetres
- A joint effusion will commonly coexist with a full-thickness tear and joint fluid will pass then into the subacromial subdeltoid bursa
- Degenerative change of the AC joint and impingement changes in the greater tuberosity are common accompaniments

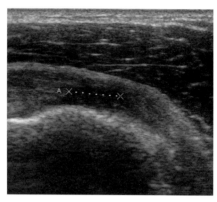

Fig. 4.18 Ultrasound showing a supraspinatus full-thickness tear.

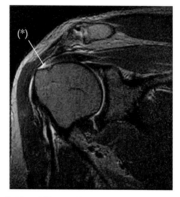

Fig. 4.19 Coronal oblique MR image shows a small tear at the insertion of supraspinatus tendon(*).

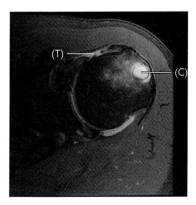

Fig. 4.20 Subscapularis tear(T) and intra-osseous cyst(C).

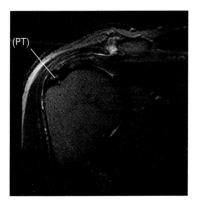

Fig. 4.21 There is a partial thickness tear of the supraspinatus tendon, on a background of severe tendonosis(PT). Degenerative change is also seen in the AC joint.

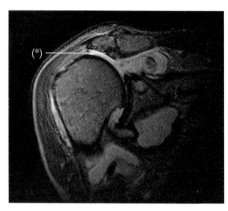

Fig. 4.22 There is complete rupture of the supraspinatus and infraspinatus tendons, and the humeral head abuts the under surface of the acromion(*).

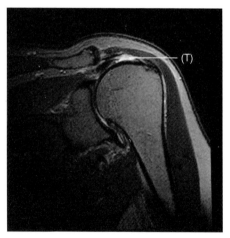

Fig. 4.23 MR of the shoulder shows there is some retraction (around 2cm)(T).

Cuff calcification

Calcific tendonitis refers to a specific condition in which the tendons of the rotator cuff, most commonly supraspinatus, are affected by calcium hydroxyapatite deposition which usually subsequently resorbs. It is possible that the inflammation associated with the resorption phase is responsible for the severe pain characterizing the condition. However, asymptomatic calcification within the cuff is a relatively frequent radiographic finding and the relationship of this finding to symptoms is not always clear cut.

Clinical features

- Usually affects those between 30–60 years of age
- Rapid onset severe, diffuse pain in the shoulder occasionally with systemic symptoms (e.g. fever, anorexia)
- No history of preceding trauma
- Constant discomfort with difficulty sleeping (night pain is prominent)
- Localized tenderness is common and pronounced
- Inability to mobilize the shoulder normally due to pain (especially abduction)
- Impingement is invariable
- In the acute stage the arm may be held in internal rotation
- A painful arc is often present
- In chronic cases, wasting of the supraspinatus may be visible

Imaging modalities

Radiography

- This is the best technique for demonstrating calcific tendonitis
- The diagnosis is made by demonstrating calcium in the rotator cuff tendons
- This is clearly visible on plain films of the shoulder
- Calcium may however be absent in early disease
- Discrete deposits of uniform intensity or a fluffy appearance is seen depending upon stage of disease

A plain film of the shoulder is extremely worthwhile in cases of fairly sudden onset shoulder pain to exclude calcific tendonitis (Fig. 4.24).

Ultrasound (US)

- Ultrasound detects calcific tendonitis well
- The calcium is seen as an area of echogenicity within the tendon and its size can be assessed accurately
- Ultrasound can also be used to guide needle interventions if appropriate

Magnetic resonance imaging (MRI)

- MRI relies on the presence of protons, and therefore is not good at detecting abnormalities of calcification generally
- When seen, the calcific tendonitis is seen as an area of signal void (i.e. black) (Fig. 4.25)
- Cuff tears do not coexist with calcific tendonitis as otherwise the calcium would be dispersed

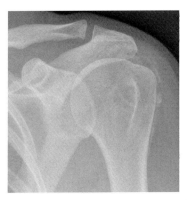

Fig. 4.24 Frontal plain film shows that calcium is seen in the subacromial subdeltoid bursa. This has arisen from calcific tendonitis of the supraspinatus tendon which has burst into the bursa, as part of its natural history.

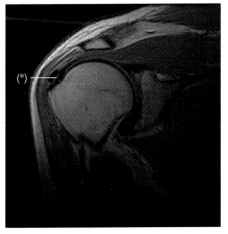

Fig. 4.25 Coronal oblique proton density-weighted image shows a dense area of low signal(*).

Internal impingement

Internal impingement results from pinching of the humeral tuberosity against the glenoid labrum. It is a common cause of posterior shoulder pain in the throwing or overhead athlete.

Clinical features

- Occurs predominantly in young adults
- Insidious onset
- No history of trauma
- Posterior shoulder pain is associated primarily with athletic or overhead activity (especially throwing)
- Stiffness of the shoulder may be present
- Associated with anterior instability
- Limitation of internal rotation
- Secondary rotator cuff tendinopathy may develop

Imaging modalities

Radiography
- This is usually normal

Ultrasound (US)
- Cannot image intra-articular structures, and therefore no abnormality is seen.

Magnetic resonance imaging (MRI)
- A variety of abnormalities can be seen with the main changes relating to tears and irregularity of the posterior superior labrum (Fig. 4.26).

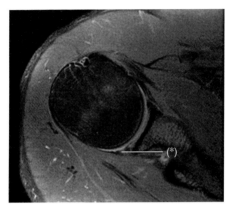

Fig. 4.26 Axial MR arthrogram. A tear of the posterior superior labrum as a result of internal impingement(*).

Subacromial impingement

Subacromial impingement occurs when anatomical structures are trapped between the humeral head and the under surface of the acromion, AC joint and coraco–acromial ligament. This most commonly involves the supraspinatus tendon and subacromial bursa.

Predisposing factors leading to impingement:
- Down-sloping or hook-like acromion
- Acromioclavicular osteophytes
- Acromial spur.
- Muscle imbalance, cuff weakness
- Instability
- Overhead workers

Clinical

- This is the commonest clinical syndrome of those presenting with shoulder pain
- Occurs at any age, usually >40 years
- Onset may be acute or chronic
- Pain felt in shoulder region
- Night pain due to lying on shoulder may be prominent
- Active and passive movements may be limited by pain
- A painful arc (60–120°) is common and the pain may be eradicated following a subacromial injection of local anaesthetic

Impingement may be assessed by forcing the affected arm in pronation into full anterior flexion thereby placing the rotator cuff against the under-side of the anterior acromion (Neer's test).

Another test involves placing the arm into 90° of abduction and flexed to 30° with the examiner supporting the patient's flexed elbow. With the other hand the examiner holds the patients shoulder girdle whilst forcibly internally rotating and elevating the affected arm (Hawkins–Kennedy test).

The subacromial bursa may become inflamed, thickened, and then scarred in subacromial impingement. Furthermore impingement may lead to supraspinatus tendinopathy.

Imaging modalities

Radiography

- Degenerative change of the AC joint
- Irregularity of the under surface of the acromion
- Degenerative change of the greater tuberosity
- On the axial view, the anterior process of the acromion may be elongated—'anterior spur'

Ultrasound (US)

- Ultrasound may be normal, but usually demonstrates some damage to the cuff tendons and/or bursitis

Magnetic resonance imaging (MRI)

Corresponding to the plain film findings, the features will be:
- Degenerative change of the AC joint, which indents the superior surface of the supraspinatus tendon (Fig. 4.27 and 4.28)

- An os acromiale may be present
- An impingement cyst may be seen in the humeral head
- Careful assessment of the cuff is needed to detect associated cuff tears
- There may be fluid in the subacromial or subdeltoid bursae

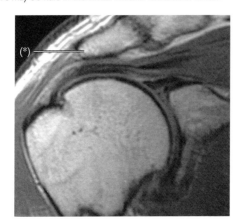

Fig. 4.27 Coronal oblique MR shows degenerative change of the right AC joint, but the impingement is largely due to the slope of the acromion laterally which narrows the subacromial space(*).

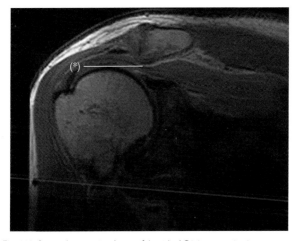

Fig. 4.28 Severe degenerative change of the right AC joint causes impingement on the superior surface of the underlying supraspinatus tendon(*).

Adhesive capsulitis (frozen shoulder)

Adhesive capsulitis is one of the most enigmatic conditions in medicine. The aetiology is unknown, however macroscopically the capsule becomes thickened and contracted.

Typically it passes through three phases:
- Freezing phase: painful shoulder with reduced mobility
- Frozen phase: immobile shoulder with pain slowly dissipating
- Thawing phase: return of shoulder movement

The whole process may take more than three years to resolve

Associated conditions
- Rotator cuff tendinopathy
- Diabetes mellitus
- Thyroid disease
- Immobility (e.g. stroke)
- Following acute myocardial infarct AMI and stroke
- Chronic regional pain syndrome (CRPS) type 1 (secondary to capsulitis)

Clinical
- Those aged between 40–70, women > men
- Onset may be acute, subacute or chronic
- A history of trauma (often mild) may be evident
- Pain felt diffusely and deeply in shoulder
- Night pain may be severe
- Wasting may develop following prolonged immobility
- Globally reduced active and passive movement
- Assessment of the rotator cuff and impingement is difficult due to the pain and immobility

Imaging modalities
Radiography
- The radiographs are usually normal
- The only way to diagnose adhesive capsulitis radiologically is with arthrography (Fig. 4.29). Contrast medium is injected into the joint and the following signs are seen:
  - The injection is painful
  - Only a small amount of fluid can be injected (typically 5mls)
  - The capsular insertion is irregular
  - Lymphatic filling may be present (Fig. 4.30)
  - During the injection, the syringe refills if the thumb is taken off the plunger during the procedure

Ultrasound (US)
- Normal in adhesive capsulitis

Magnetic resonance imaging (MRI)
- Usually normal, although some authors report enhancement around the joint if contrast medium is given intravenously

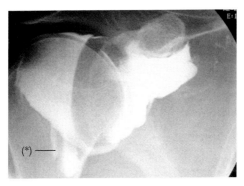

Fig. 4.29 Arthrogram of the shoulder showing a tight joint with fluid filling the biceps tendon sheath, a small subglenoid recess, and irregularity of the capsular insertion(*).

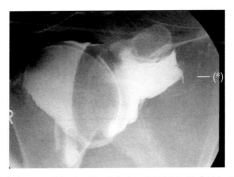

Fig. 4.30 Arthrogram of the shoulder displaying a tight joint with fluid, having been forced into the lymphatics, tracking medially from the subcoracoid bursa(*).

Biceps tendon lesions

Biceps tendon lesions may occur in isolation or associated with rotator cuff pathology. The spectrum of biceps tendon lesions include:
- tendonitis/tenosynovitis
- tendinosis
- various degrees of tear (partial, full thickness and rupture)
- instability in the bicipital groove (subluxation or dislocation)

Clinical features
- Biceps tendon lesions occur at any age, however rupture usually develops in those >40 years
- Pain in the region of the tendon may come on acutely or insidiously although rupture may not cause pain
- A history of trauma may be evident with subluxation, dislocation, and ruptures
- Night pain is not particularly prominent
- Tenderness may be present over the tendon in the bicipital groove
- Weakness may be present with tears
- If the long head of biceps is ruptured then the characteristic Popeye sign may develop (the belly of biceps appears prominent and globular in the lower third of the arm)
- Snapping of the tendon over the anterior shoulder may occur
- Chronic subluxation may lead to tendinopathy and tear due to attrition

It is worth noting that the bicipital tendon is often tender where it lies in its groove in normal individuals.

Imaging modalities
Radiography
- Other than irregularity in relation to the bicipital groove, which may be associated with bicipital tendinosis, plain film findings will be normal

Ultrasound (US)
An excellent technique for evaluating the biceps tendon.

Tendinosis will be seen as:
- Swelling of the tendon
- Hypoechogenicity
- Irregularity or inhomogeneity of the tendon

A partial thickness tear may be seen by
- Longitudinal fissures within the tendon

A full thickness tear will be seen as:
- A torn tendon with retracted into the upper arm

Ultrasound is also good for determining a tendon that is subluxed medially

Magnetic resonance imaging (MRI)
- MRI is accurate at determining tendinosis, partial and full-thickness tears of the biceps tendon
- Can detect subluxation by the abnormal location of the tendon (Fig. 4.31)

- In tendinosis, the tendon is swollen, oedematous and may be heterogeneous (Fig. 4.32)
- Longitudinal fissures and partial tears are seen as areas of longitudinal high signal within the tendon on the fluid-sensitive sequence
- In subluxation or bicipital tendon tear, the bicipital groove will be empty
- When subluxation is present, the tendon will be seen lying medial to the groove
- Subluxation is usually associated with damage to the subscapularis

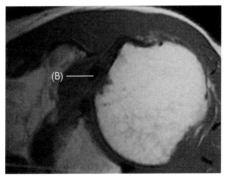

Fig. 4.31 Axial T1-weighted image shows medial subluxation of the biceps tendon (B).

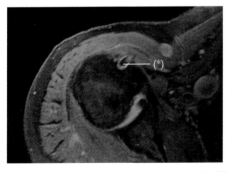

Fig. 4.32 Tendinosis of the biceps tendon is seen as high signal within it(*).

Acromioclavicular joint trauma

AC joint trauma is common especially amongst athletes (e.g. rugby and Australian Rules football). The joint may be sprained/strained or it may sublux or dislocate.

Clinical features
- May occur at any age
- Onset of pain is acute following trauma
- Symptoms are worse with movement and with certain activities such as lifting and carrying heavy objects
- Night pain is common
- Clicking may occur
- There is no weakness
- There may be associated instability
- The pain can be well localized (often a finger can be placed on the joint to indicate the site of pain)
- Deformity suggests subluxation or dislocation
- A high arc of pain may be present
- Full active and passive movement may be limited by pain

Imaging modalities
Radiography (Fig. 4.33)
- Subluxation of the AC joint is best appreciated on plain films
- The relation of the outer end of clavicle to the acromion is seen best on the frontal radiograph, and the degree of damage can be staged depending on the findings
- In the normal situation, the inferior end of the acromion and the clavicle are at the same level
- A complete dislocation is seen when the under-surface of the clavicle is higher than the superior surface of the acromion
- Subluxation occurs when the outer end of the clavicle is cranially migrated but not to the extent that it is higher than the superior surface of the acromion

Ultrasound (US)
- Ultrasound has no role in this context

Magnetic resonance imaging (MRI)
- Not needed to diagnose AC joint trauma, as plain films suffice
- If an MR is performed then it will show bone marrow oedema on either side of the joint acutely, which will settle in approximately six months
- Otherwise the findings mirror the plain film findings

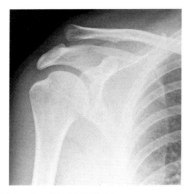

Fig. 4.33 Total dislocation of the right AC joint.

Acromioclavicular joint arthritis

AC joint arthritis is relatively common and may occur as part of generalized osteoarthritis. A history of previous injury may well predispose to its development.

Clinical features

- Older age groups
- Chronic onset of pain in the region of the joint
- Night pain may be prominent and patients have difficulty sleeping on the affected side
- Overhead activities may be restricted
- Clicking can occur
- There is no weakness
- Instability may be present
- Swelling and deformity may be evident and is often tender
- A superior arc of pain is often present
- Full active and passive movement may be limited by pain

Secondary rotator cuff tendinopathy may develop with ACJ OA.

Patients are very good at localizing AC joint pain and are usually able to place a finger directly on the affected area.

AC joint symptoms commonly occur as a result of instability (assess anteroposterior and inferosuperior laxity).

Imaging modalities

Radiography

- Plain films only show the bony components of the joint
- May show osteophytes on the superior or inferior portion of the joint margin

Ultrasound (US)

- Although the superior osteophytes will be visible, ultrasound has no particular role in this context

Magnetic resonance imaging (MRI) (Figs. 4.34, 4.35)

- In addition to the bony changes seen on plain films, MR will also show the soft tissue thickening commonly associated with this condition
- MR will also demonstrate any associated damage to the underlying cuff tendons

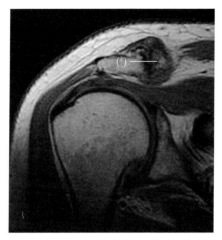

Fig. 4.34 MR of the shoulder shows bulbous degenerative change of the right AC joint(*).

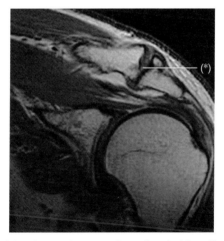

Fig. 4.35 Moderately severe degenerative change affects the AC joint(*).

Investigating hand and wrist problems

Anatomy

Bony

The bones of the wrist consist of the distal radius and ulna, the proximal row of carpal bones and the distal row. The radius and ulna articulate with each other, allowing for some rotation, and with the proximal carpal row. The proximal row consists of the scaphoid, lunate, and triquetrum with the pisiform as a sesamoid bone in the tendon of flexor carpi ulnaris. The distal row consists of the trapezium, trapezoid, capitate, and hamate. A way to help differentiate trapezium from trapezoid is that thumb (which articulates with the trapezium) rhymes with trapezium.

The joints of the wrist are the radiocarpal joint, the midcarpal joint and the carpo–metacarpal joints. The joint spaces can be demonstrated with arthrography. The radio and ulno carpal compartment should not communicate with the other wrist joint compartments. If it does during arthrography it implies damage to the intercarpal ligaments. The mid carpal joint often normally communicates with the carpo–metacarpal joints via the trapezium–trapezoid joint.

Ligaments and triangular fibro cartilage complex (TFCC)

There are many ligaments in the wrist and most of the carpal bones are linked to each other. Tears of these ligaments can lead to symptoms and are best seen by MR arthrography. One of the most important ligaments is the scapho-lunate ligament. Rupture of this ligament causes a wide scapholunate distance known either as the Terry Thomas, Letterman or Madonna sign.

The TFCC is a complex structure which supports the distal radio ulnar joint. It acts like the meniscus in the knee and transmits and distributes some of the forces in the wrist. Damage to the TFCC can lead to pain and instability of the ulnar aspect of the wrist. Assessment of the TFCC is best achieved by MR arthrography. An important part of the arthrogram is the injection under fluoroscopy. Carefully watching where the contrast goes and when can help accurately detection of ligamentous injuries.

The extensor tendons at the wrist are divided into six separate fibrous compartments each containing a variable number of tendons contained with a synovial sheath. These are numbered 1 to 6 from the radial side of the wrist.

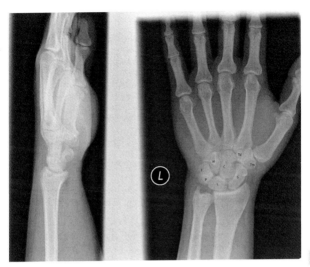

Fig. 5.1 Normal plain film of the wrist showing the carpal bones. S, scaphoid; L, lunate; T, triquetrum; P, pisiform; H, hamate; C, capitate, Td, trapezoid; Tm, trapezium.

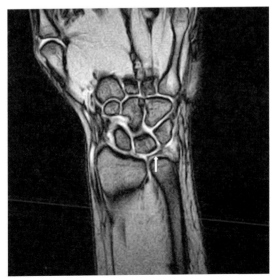

Fig. 5.2 MRI of a normal wrist showing the meniscal appearance of the TFCC (arrow).

Wrist instability

Stability of the wrist is provided by the complex arrangement of the individual carpal bones. These bones are divided into proximal and distal rows held together by the ligamentous interconnections that guide and constrain movement of one bone on another.

Most of the axial load applied to the wrist is borne by the radius and lateral carpal bones, and consequently, there is a high frequency of injury to distal radius, scaphoid and its ligamentous attachments.

Carpal instability results from two possible mechanisms:

- Dynamic instability with rupture or attenuation of intrinsic and extrinsic carpal ligaments with normal alignment of bones at rest but lost under movement and applied load.
- Static instability occurs with malalignment of the carpal or radiocarpal bones.

Numerous instabilities have been described including midcarpal instability, dorsal intercalated segment instability (DISI) and volar intercalated segment instability (VISI).

The intercalated segment referred to in these descriptions is the proximal row of carpal bones. They are termed intercalated as there are no tendon attachments onto these bones: as such they have no active movement of their own and act as a buffer between the distal carpal row and the radius and ulna. Damage to the extrinsic ligaments that support the proximal row or to the intrinsic ligaments linking them together thus has a dramatic effect on the proximal carpal row function.

Midcarpal instability involves dissociation or subluxation of the capitate and the hamate on the lunate and triquetrum respectively. The pattern of dislocation and instability describes the direction in which the lunate rotates and the proximal row of carpal bones collapses due to laxity.

In VISI, the distal aspect of the lunate rotates volarly as a result of instability of extrinsic carpal ligaments. VISI deformity is seen in association with inflammatory arthropathies such as rheumatoid or pyrophosphate arthropathy and disruption of the triquetrolunate ligament.

In DISI, the distal aspect of the lunate rotates dorsally as a result of instability of laxity of the scapholunate ligaments. These are readily demonstrated in the neutral lateral wrist radiographs (Fig. 5.3). The normal angle between the scaphoid and the lunate is 30–60°. DISI deformity is seen in patients with scapholunate ligament disruption and in patients with inflammatory arthropathy.

Scapholunate instability

Rupture of scapholunate ligament occurs frequently in sports and trauma with or without associated fracture. Scapholunate dissociation is the most common instability of the wrist. Injury usually occurs following a fall on the outstretched hand with the wrist extended and an axial force applied to the base of the palm. This leads to progressive flexion posture of the scaphoid and displacement of lunate to adopt a DISI pattern.

An anteroposterior (AP) radiograph (supinated view of the wrist with maximal ulnar deviation while gripping) may show widening of the scapholunate space beyond 3mm—known as Terry Thomas sign. MRI with contrast or arthroscopy may confirm complete disrupted scapholunate ligaments (Fig. 5.4). Surgery with ligamentous repair may be required.

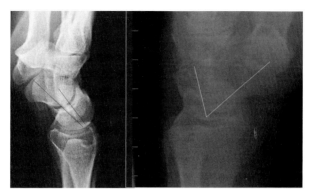

Fig. 5.3 Wrist instability. The angle between the scaphoid and the lunate is less than 30° on the left (VISI) and more than 60° on the right (DISI).

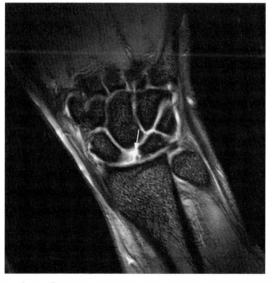

Fig. 5.4 Coronal T2-weighted image demonstrates disruption of the scapholunate ligament (arrow) with widening of the scapholunate interval.

Wrist ligament injury

Dorsal and supination forces are likely to produce perilunate injuries whilst palmar and pronation forces are likely to involve the ulnar side of the wrist. A torn ligament is suspected when the patient reports pain that is out of proportion to the injury.

The triangular fibrocartilage complex

Ulnar wrist pain and weakness caused by a fall onto a pronated out-stretched hand may suggest an injury to the triangular fibrocartilage complex (TFCC), which stabilizes the distal radioulnar joint and cushions the ulnar carpus.

Tenderness immediately distal in the hollow between the pisiform and ulnar styloid usually indicates a TFCC injury. This injury may also be tested with McMurray's manoeuvre in which the triquetrum is manipulated against the head of the ulna with the wrist in ulnar deviation, with palpable crepitus or snap.

Plain radiographs may demonstrate ulnar variance and degenerative changes. MRI is highly useful to demonstrate TFCC injuries (Fig. 5.5) and to assess the surrounding tissues eg disruption of the extensor car-piulnaris tendon sheath and ulnotriquetral ligament.

Distal radioulnar joint

- This joint is stabilized by the joint capsule, the interosseous membrane, TFCC, the pronator quadratus and forearm muscles. The radius dislocates relative to the ulna but the injury is described in relation to the ulna's position.
- Dorsal dislocation of the distal radioulnar (DRU) joint is common and results from a fall onto a pronated hand. It involves disruption of the dorsal radioulnar ligament of the TFCC and dorsal capsule of DRU joint.
- Volar dislocation of the joint usually results from a forced supination injury or direct blow to the dorsum of the forearm.

Radiology may suggest features of instability with widening of radioulnar joint and dislocation. An accurate lateral view is required for diagnosis.

An ulnar styloid fracture with detachment of the ulnar styloid process from the shaft may result in destabilization of the DRUJ.

A CT scan may be required to confirm the diagnosis as lateral radiographs can be misleading as a result of rotation. Checking the radial styloid lies at the midpoint of the radial articular surface on the lateral view is a good way to confirm the lateral view of the wrist is a 'true' lateral. MR can also demonstrate subluxation and/or dislocation of the DRUJ in the axial plane of imaging.

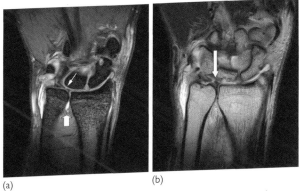

(a)   (b)

Fig. 5.5 Triangular fibrocartilage perforation. (a) MRI Coronal T2-weighted image demonstrates a tear in the TFCC (small arrow) and contrast in the DRUJ (thick arrow); (b) shows the same TFCC with T1-weighted images.

Scaphoid fractures

Scaphoid fractures are common and frequently result from falling on an outstretched hand. Scaphoid fractures are of concern because the blood supply of the scaphoid is from distal to proximal. A fracture through the waist of the scaphoid can result in non-union which may result in the proximal portion becoming necrotic. This in turn can lead to disabling arthritis. If treated early this complication can be avoided.

The most common site of fracture is the waist (60–70%) followed by the distal pole (approx 20%). Due to the blood supply the distal fractures have a better prognosis.

The rate of necrosis post scaphoid fracture is 10–15%.

Other carpal fractures and ligamentous injury are associated with scaphoid fractures and should be considered.

Treatment of scaphoid fractures depends on the location and type. Distal pole fractures are normally treated conservatively unless there is significant displacement. 90% of non-displaced waist fractures will unite with immobilization. Other factors are taken into account when deciding on management. Displaced waist fractures require fixation as do proximal fractures. The different types of fixation are outside the scope of this text.

Imaging modalities

Radiography

Imaging is based on clinical suspicion. Plain 'scaphoid views' should detect many scaphoid fractures (Fig 5.6). Imaging of the occult scaphoid fractures is controversial and partly determined by local availibility of imaging. Repeat plain films after 10–14 days can detect fractures. Immediate CT is excellent at showing bony anatomy and can accurately show any displacement.

Magnetic resonance imaging (MRI)

MRI can show linear high signal through the scaphoid even when fractures are undisplaced and is considered the gold standard for occult fracture detection.

When a fracture has been diagnosed and the viability of the proximal pole is threatened MRI can assess fragment viability. Without contrast high signal in the proximal pole on T1- and T2-weighted imaging implies viability (Fig. 5.7). If the proximal pole enhances after gadolinium contrast then it is viable.

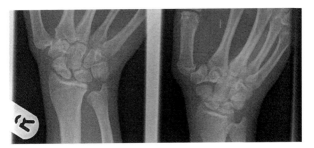

Fig. 5.6 Plain film shows a fracture through the waist of the scaphoid.

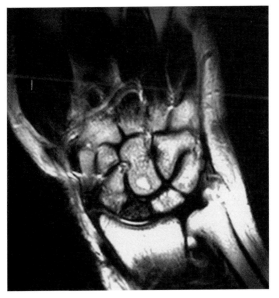

Fig. 5.7 Low signal of the proximal pole of the scaphoid implies that the proximal pole is non-viable.

Other wrist fractures

The most common fractures of the wrist are fractures of the distal radius and ulna. These are normally caused by falling on an outstretched hand. There are various eponyms for different types of fracture. The most common are Colles, Smith's and Barton's. What is more important than the name of the fracture is whether the injury involves the articular surface and how many parts it is in? These facts are important for prognostication, management, and surgical planning.

- Ligamentous and TFCC injuries can accompany distal radial fractures in up to 50% of cases.
- The Galeazzi fracture is a combination of a radial fracture and dislocation of the distal radioulnar joint (Fig. 5.8).
- Carpal bones other than the scaphoid can be fractured. The triquetrum can be fractured either by direct force or the dorsal surface can be fractured by contact with the ulnar or dorsal ligament avulsion. This latter fracture is often seen on plain film as a flake of bone dorsally on the lateral view.
- Hamate fractures can be problematic due to the relation of the hook of the hamate to other structures. Fractures of the hook can lead to osteonecrosis and median or ulnar nerve problems. These fractures can be caused by impaction sports injury: in racket sports this affects the dominant hand and in golf the non-dominant hand.
- Isolated fractures of the capitate, lunate, pisiform, trapezium, and trapezoid are rare.
- Combinations of carpal fractures in these bones are more common and tend to occur in association with fracture dislocations. The reason for this is the complex nature of the intracarpal ligaments. One association of note is fractures of the scaphoid with concurrent fractures of the capitate and triquetrum. This fracture pattern is unstable and needs to be recognized.

Imaging modalities

Radiography

Most fractures in the wrist can be diagnosed on plain film but some of the more complex or unusual patterns may require CT for surgical planning (Fig. 5.9).

Computed tomography (CT)

CT 3D reconstructions can also help with surgical planning in the more complex cases.

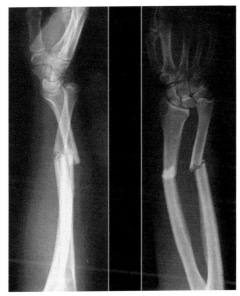

Fig. 5.8 Plain radiograph of a fracture of the radius and ulna. The fractures are both displaced.

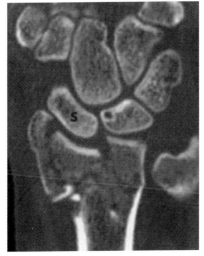

Fig. 5.9 Coronal CT reconstruction of a comminuted distal radial fracture involving the articular surface.

Fracture dislocations of the wrist

Dislocation of the radioulnar joint in the wrist is uncommon and is normally associated with a fracture of the radius. This is a Galeazzi fracture. There are different types of Galeazzi fracture, the most common of which is a fracture of the radial shaft with ulna dislocation at the wrist.

Any bone of the carpus can dislocate but isolated dislocations are rare. Certain patterns of dislocation occur because of the strength of some of the carpal ligaments and the shape of the radio-carpal joint. Two common patterns are the lunate and perilunate dislocation.

Perilunate dislocation

Hyperextension forces can transmit through the radius and into the carpi. The radius tends to hold the lunate in place due to the cup shape of its articular surface. With increasing force the capitate and other carpal bones can dislocate leaving the lunate in place articulating with the distal radius. This is a perilunate dislocation (Fig. 5.10). The key to differentiating between a lunate and perilunate dislocation is asking the question: 'is the lunate in the right place?'.

Lunate dislocation

The lunate can be forced ventrally creating a lunate subluxation (Fig. 5.11) or frank dislocation. In this injury the capitate may migrate proximally and line up with the radius on a lateral view with the lunate tilted, often by as much as 90°.

Imaging modalities

Radiography

Fracture dislocations of the wrist can best appreciated radiographically by assessing the arcs of the carpus on the PA view. The lesser and greater arcs involve the distal and proximal articular surfaces of the triquetral, lunate, and scaphoid respectively. Disruption of the smooth curve of lines drawn along these articular surfaces should raise the possibility of lunate and perilunate dislocations. Careful scrutiny of the lateral view will then be required to look at lunate capitate and radius relations.

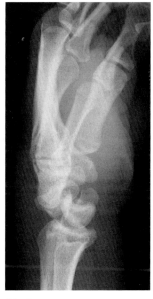

Fig. 5.10 Perilunate dislocation.

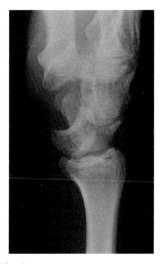

Fig. 5.11 Lunate dislocation.

Arthritis of the wrist

This may be classified as degenerative, inflammatory (rheumatoid arthritis, crystal arthropathy) or traumatic conditions.

Osteoarthritis

Osteoarthritis (OA) can affect the wrist and usually affects the first carpometacarpal, scaphotrapezoid, and pisiform–triquetral articulations in nodular generalized OA. Wrist OA can be secondary to fractures and disorders such as Keinboch's disease (osteonecrosis of the lunate) or hamatolunate impingement.

Crystal arthropathy/calcium pyrophosphate dihydrate arthropathy (CPPD)

Also known as pseudogout, the diagnosis is confirmed with demonstration of distinctive crystals in the synovial fluid. These patients present with an acute usually monoarthritis that is extremely painful, the differential diagnosis clinically is often infection or true gout.

Plain radiographs may reveal chondrocalcinosis in the triangular cartilage of the wrist (Fig. 5.12). Advanced scapholunate collapse with indentation in the distal radius by scaphoid bone may be present. This may be associated with prominent exuberant osteophyte and cyst formation. Erosive changes may be detected around the distal inferior radioulnar and radiocarpal joints. VISI or DISI deformities may well be present.

Several metabolic conditions including haemachromatosis and hyperparathyroidism may promote premature CPPD deposition. These may be screened with serum calcium, magnesium, phosphate, iron, measurement of iron-binding capacity, and alkaline phosphatase.

Rheumatoid arthritis

- Erosion and swelling around the ulnar styloid process are early signs of rheumatoid arthritis (RA).
- Similar changes may occur over the distal radius, triquetrum, and pisiform.
- Progressive disease will ultimately lead to shortening of the wrist, scapholunate dissociation, carpal supination, translocation of the carpus in a ulnar and volar direction, radial deviation of the carpus, and dorsal subluxation of the ulna (Fig. 5.13).

Imaging modalities

Magnetic resonance imaging (MRI)

MRI of the wrist may demonstrate bone erosions, synovial hypertrophy, synovitis/pannus, and tenosynovitis. It may reveal other features of tendinitis, enthesitis, ligament and tendon tears, bone marrow oedema, and joint effusions.

Ultrasound

Ultrasound can be of value in demonstrating effusion, synovitis, and erosion, and has been shown to be more sensitive and accurate than clinical examination. It can also guide needle placement for intraarticular therapy.

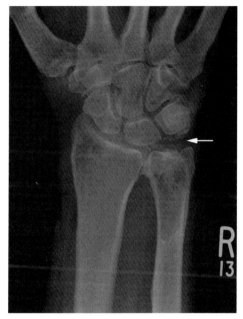

Fig. 5.12 Chondrocalcinosis is seen in the triangular fibrocartilage (arrow).

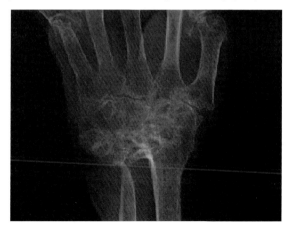

Fig. 5.13 Radiograph of left wrist demonstrates marked destructive erosive changes and joint space narrowing in a pancarpal distribution with resorption of the distal ulna.

Wrist ganglia

Ganglia are cystic swellings containing jelly-like fluid under tension. They more commonly affect women in the third to fifth decades. They always communicate with an adjacent tendon sheath, joint or ligament.

Common sites include dorsally from the scapholunate ligament, the radial aspect of the radioscaphoid and midcarpal joints and seed ganglia arising on the flexor tendon sheaths of the fingers. The aetiology is unclear but may represent remodelling of the fibrous capsule of the joint.

Most disappear spontaneously but occasionally, they may result in neural compression. The deep branch of the ulnar nerve may be compressed by a ganglion in Guyon's canal. The radial artery may be compromised by a ganglion arising from the trapezioscaphoid joint.

Imaging modalities

Radiographs

Usually uninformative, but a large lesion can appear as a soft-tissue mass lacking calcifications. Occasionally compression on adjacent bones can be detected.

Magnetic resonance imaging (MRI)

Ganglia usually have homogenous signal with well-defined margins. They are isointense to muscle on T1-weighted sequences and hyperintense on T2-weighted sequences. There is no contrast enhancement.

Ultrasound (US)

Demonstrates a well-defined anechoic structure close to a joint with posterior acoustic enhancement, consistent with its cystic nature (Fig. 5.14).

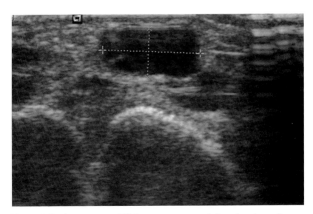

Fig. 5.14 Ganglion: transverse US demonstrates an anechoic oval cystic ganglion without a definitive wall with posterior acoustic enhancement in the dorsal compartment.

Tendon anatomy of the wrist

Flexor tendons

The tendons of the wrist are best examined using ultrasound. Tendons can be traced to their insertions using this method. The flexor tendons are split into four groups.

The most ulnar tendon is flexor carpi ulnaris. This can be seen inserting into the pisiform and hamate. Next are the tendons in the carpal tunnel. These tendons are flexor digitorum superficialis and profundus. These can be traced distally to each digit.

On the radial side of the carpal tunnel are flexor pollicis longus (FPL) which can be best appreciated by scanning while flexing and extending the thum. Flexor carpi radialis lies outside of the carpal tunnel on the anterior aspect of the roof and can be traced to its insertion in the 2nd and 3rd metacarpals.

Extensor tendons

The extensor tendons (Fig. 5.15) are divided into six compartments:
- *Extensor pollicis brevis* and **abductor pollicis longus.** These tendons are clinically important as they are inflamed in De Quervain's tenosynovitis and they form the lateral border of the anatomical snuff box.
- *Extensor carpi radialis brevis* and **longus.** The brevis is on the ulnar side. They insert into the third and second metacarpals respectively.
- *Extensor pollicis longus.* This is divided from compartment 2 by Lister's bony tubercle which can be felt on the back of the wrist. This is the dorsal border of the anatomical snuff box.
- *Extensors to the fingers.* The indicis tendon is deep to the other four.
- *Extensor digit minimi.* The little finger has two extensor tendons. They join at the metacarpal–phalangeal joint.
- *Extensor carpi ulnaris.* This inserts into the base of the 5th metacarpal.

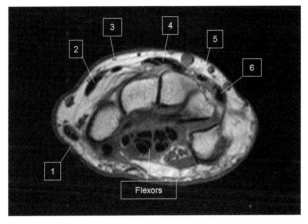

Fig. 5.15 Axial T₁ MRI showing the tendon compartments.

Finger tenosynovitis

Tenosynovitis is a common inflammatory process of the hand and is usually as a result of repetitive activities and sport. However, this can also occur in systemic inflammatory joint disease such as rheumatoid arthritis.

During the acute stage, there is an accumulation of peritendinous fluid and thickening of the tendon. In the chronic stage, there is thickening of the tendon and synovial sheaths with formation of cysts and nodules.

Clinically, flexor tenosynovitis is present if passive flexion of a finger exceeds active flexion. Crepitus may be palpated over the palm as the fingers are extended and flexed.

Imaging modalities

Ultrasound (US)

Ultrasound demonstrates synovial thickening and sheath effusion as hypoechoic regions surrounding the echogenic tendon. Power Doppler can distinguish thickened synovium from fluid by depicting flow which is present in the synovium and not effusion (Fig. 5.16). Aspiration of fluid and steroid injection may be performed if required.

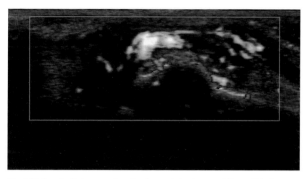

Fig. 5.16 Longitudinal power Doppler demonstrates increased flow within the tendon sheath indicating inflammation of the right index finger.

Carpal tunnel syndrome

This is an entrapment neuropathy caused by the compression of the median nerve in the fibroosseous carpal tunnel. Focal demyelination or Wallerian degeneration can develop with progression of disease resulting in functional impairment of the thumb and hand.

Conditions associated with carpal tunnel syndrome (CTS):

- Pregnancy
- Diabetes mellitus
- Myxoedema
- Systemic sclerosis
- Rheumatoid arthritis
- Previous wrist trauma
- Myeloma
- Amyloid
- Acromegaly

Sensory symptoms typically precede motor impairment with painful paraesthesia over the fingers and hands. The symptoms may awaken the patient from sleep with an attempt to rub their hands together or shake the fingers to relieve the symptoms. The symptoms may be aggravated in certain positions and activities such as driving or lifting. Hanging the hand down or changing position usually eases the symptoms.

There may be no abnormal signs although with more severe disease the thenar eminence may appear wasted, particularly over the abductor pollicis brevis, and some sensory changes may occur over the tips of the thumb, index, middle, and radial aspect of the ring fingers.

Special clinical tests to look for Phalen and Tinel signs are often used but not sufficiently sensitive to support the diagnosis of carpal tunnel syndrome.

Clinical features

The diagnosis is usually suspected clinically.

Nerve conduction studies (NCS) in early compression will show a diminished response in the size of the sensory action potentials with delay seen first in the median palmar branches. Over time, there may be absence of the median sensory action potentials, prolonged distal motor latencies and even signs of denervation in abductor pollicis brevis. Predisposing causes for CTS should be investigated.

Carpal tunnel syndrome can also be diagnosed with US or MRI by demonstrating an increase in the cross-sectional area of the median nerve at the level of the pisiform bone (Figs 5.17 and 5.18).

This may be managed conservatively with splinting and activity modification. Local steroid injection and decompressive surgery may be considered if these measures fail to alleviate symptoms or in those with progressive motor dysfunction.

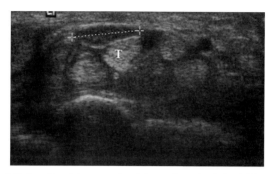

Fig. 5.17 Carpal tunnel: transverse view of the carpal tunnel at the level of the pisiform demonstrates flattening of the median nerve (line) superficial to the flexor digitorum tendons (T).

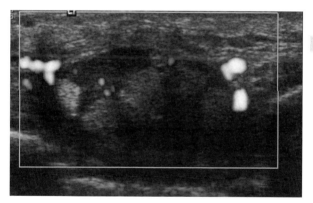

Fig. 5.18 The median nerve is flat due to extensive tenosynovitis as shown with power Doppler.

Wrist ulnar neuropathy

This is far less common than ulnar nerve neuropathy at the elbow. Pure motor neuropathies are the most common (>50%), followed by mixed sensory and motor (≈33%), and most rarely, pure sensory lesions.

The superficial location of the ulnar nerve predisposes it to blunt trauma or compression. It may also be compressed as it traverses through the narrow Guyon's canal. The tunnel is bordered medially by the flexor carpi ulnaris tendon and the pisiform, anteriorly by the superficial part of the flexor retinaculum, and posteriorly by the flexor retinaculum.

The most common cause of ulnar neuropathy at the wrist is repetitive trauma related to occupation or misuse (e.g. cyclists) leading to oedema and inflammation of tissues within the Guyon's canal and compression of the deep terminal branch distal to the supply of the hypothenar eminence. Other possible compressive causes include ganglia, neuroma, carpal bone fractures (fracture of hamate in golfers), ulnar artery disease, anomalous muscles, rheumatoid arthritis, and lipomata.

Clinical findings include:
• Focal pain and tenderness over Guyon's canal
• Positive Tinel's sign if the sensory branch is involved
• Wasting of small muscles of hand.

Clinical features

Nerve conduction studies (NCS) are used to determine the site of entrapment precisely and establish which branches are involved.

Imaging modalities

Ultrasound (US)

The nerve normally measures approximately 2mm in diameter and appears hypoechoic on US. US may demonstrate focal narrowing of the nerve at the level of the wrist and may identify any compressive cystic lesions such as ganglion.

Magnetic resonance imaging (MRI)

MRI permits a more precise topographical evaluation of the tunnel anatomy and morphological analysis of the nerve and surrounding tissues.

Hand anatomy

The tendons of the hand are divided into flexor and extensor groups.

The flexor tendons are further divided into superficial and deep (profundus) groups. The superficialis tendon (FDS) divides into two at the proximal interphalangeal joint (PIPJ) and each slip passes around FDP to insert into the base of the middle phalanx. FDP continues more distally to insert at the base of the distal phalanx.

The flexor tendons are held in place along the fingers by a series of pulleys. These pulleys are short fibrous and fibrocartilagenous bands that stop bowstringing of the tendon as it flexes. These pulleys can be seen with ultrasound and rupture or dysfunction can be demonstrated with resisted flexion scanning.

The extensor tendons of the fingers occupy extensor compartment 4 in the wrist. The extensor tendons then merge with the deep fascia beneath the subcutaneous layer to form the extensor expansion. This splits into three at the PIPJ and a middle part inserts into the base of the middle phalanx while the two lateral parts insert into the base of the distal phalanx. The little finger has its own extensor tendon (compartment 5) but also has a second slip from the extensor digitorum group. The extensor expansion also receives attachments from the interrosei and lumbricals.

Clinical features

Apart from fractures most injuries in the hands are due to avulsive injuries. The long tendon insertions are particularly prone to avulsion. This is particularly common at the extensor insertion on the base of the distal phalanx resulting in the classic 'mallet finger' deformity.

The capsular insertions of the interphalangeal joints can avulse particularly over their volar aspect. Volar plate injury is seen as a small flake of bone next to the interphalangeal joint. The ulnar collateral ligament of the thumb can be injured resulting in disabling instability (skier's or gamekeeper's thumb). This injury can be seen on ultrasound and is not normally associated with bony injury.

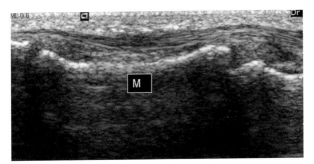

Fig. 5.19 The linear tendon is seen superficial to the middle phalanx (M). Flexor digitorum profundus can be seen inserting into the base of the distal phalanx.

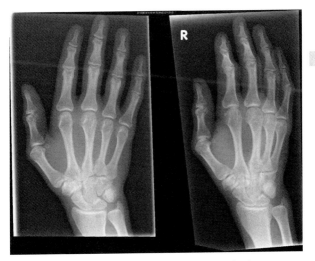

Fig. 5.20 Normal hand to compare with the arthritides later in the chapter.

Boxer's knuckle

Trauma to the metacarpophalangeal (MCP) joint may result from repetitive or isolated forceful blows with the clenched fist. Such injury usually occurs in contact sports including boxing, martial arts, and other punching sports.

The term boxer's knuckle refers to the injury sustained with damage to the sagittal bands of the extensor hood mechanism. The extensor hood overlying the MCP joint capsule comprises two distinct transversely oriented ligaments termed sagittal bands that help to stabilize the longitudinal extensor tendon during joint motion.

These ligaments are maximally stretched over the metacarpal head as a fist is formed, thus they are susceptible to injury. The radial sagittal bands are more commonly injured, producing ulnar subluxation of the tendon. Further force leads to rupture of the dorsal capsule.

Patients will notice acute pain and swelling over the radial or ulnar aspect of the MCP joint associated with loss of full joint extension due to pain and tendon subluxation. Subluxation is detected on palpation of the flexed joint associated with a popping or catching sensation.

In some cases, extensor tendon dislocation or subluxation may be difficult to assess clinically (full range of motion with no tendon subluxation or significant swelling renders palpation of the tendon difficult).

Imaging modalities

Radiography

Plain radiographs should be performed to exclude bone pathology.

Ultrasound (US)

Dynamic US with flexion and extension of the affected finger allows accurate visualization of extensor tendon subluxation or dislocation relative to the metacarpal head associated with other findings such as tenosynovitis or tendon split.

Trigger finger

Otherwise known as stenosing tenosynovitis or tendovaginitis, it describes the inflammatory changes within in the retinacular sheath and peritendinous tissue.

The site of the pathology lies in the obstruction of the first annular (A–1) pulley. The flexor tendon sheath catches as it attempts to glide through a relatively stenotic sheath, leading to impaired movement of the affected finger.

It usually affects the middle-aged and some patient groups such as those with diabetes, carpal tunnel syndrome, rheumatoid arthritis or any conditions resulting in systemic deposition of protein such as amyloidosis.

Clinical features

Usually clinical with symptomatic clicking or locking of finger or thumb. In severe cases, the finger may be locked in flexion, requiring passive manipulation of the finger into extension. In some instances, secondary contractures may occur over the PIP joints.

The patient may complain initially of painless clicking with finger movement, and may progress to painful triggering localized to the palm, MCP or PIP joints.

The ring finger and thumb are most commonly affected, with the index and small fingers being the least symptomatic. In patients with rheumatoid arthritis, palpable swelling on the palmar aspect of the affected digit may be demonstrated and rupture of the affected flexor tendon may occur in severe cases.

Non-operative treatment includes rest splinting or steroid injection into the tendon sheath. Surgical intervention may be considered when conventional treatment fails and should be considered for those who wish a quick and definitive relief.

Imaging modalities

Ultrasound (US)

These lesions are easily detected on US. Thickening of the flexor tendons, A1 pulley and synovial sheath with altered echotexture and associated peritendinous cysts on the palmar aspect of the affected metacarpophalangeal (MCP) joint may be demonstrated. There is hesitation of the thickened flexor tendon and its synovial sheath as it moves under the pulley during extension (Fig. 5.21). Dynamic longitudinal US will demonstrate the tendon catching during movement. Comparison with the contralateral unaffected digit may be helpful.

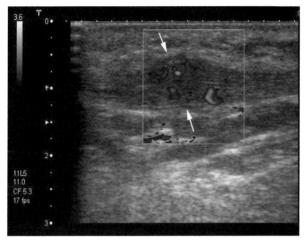

Fig. 5.21 Trigger finger: Thickened tendon (arrow) associated with inflammatory changes detected on power Doppler as the tendon passes through the tendinous sheath.

Pulley finger

Flexor pulley injuries are common among rock climbers with resultant high forces applied onto the PIP joints and the digital pulley system.

The fibrous retinacular sheath for fingers is divided into five annular (A1–A5) bands and three cruciform (C1–C3) ligaments, extends from the neck of metacarpal and ends at the distal phalanx. These span from side to side across the palmar margin of the digits to stabilize the position of the flexor tendons close to the phalanges.

These injuries usually affect the A2–A4 pulleys over the middle and ring fingers.

There is an acute onset of pain while performing a difficult move or slipping off a foothold. A loud popping noise may be noted. There may evidence of local swelling and tenderness on the palmar aspect of the injured pulley. AP and lateral radiographs should be performed to exclude fractures or palmar plate avulsion injuries and chronic overuse fractures in adolescent climbers.

Imaging modalities

Diagnostic imaging will assist accurate assessment of pulley injury in particular if clinical examination is not conclusive.

Magnetic resonance imaging (MRI)

MRI cannot directly detect the damaged pulley but the T1 sequences will demonstrate the anterior displacement of the flexor tendon from the bone and the T2 sequences will be able to distinguish tendinitis, peritendinous inflammation, intra-tendon lesions and partial ruptures. It will also provide further information on the extent and position of the flexor tendon bowstringing.

Ultrasound (US)

Dynamic ultrasound examination is increasingly used as an alternative to MRI, and is able to demonstrate:

- increased distance between flexor tendon and phalanx in extension and forced flexion as an indicator of bowstringing (Fig. 5.22)
- thickening of the flexor tendon and pulley system
- real time correlation of abnormal findings with focal tenderness.

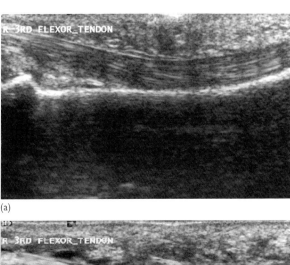

(a)

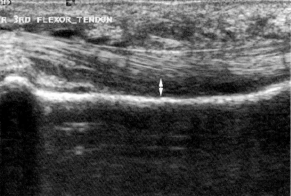

(b)

Fig. 5.22 (a) The flexor tendon is held down with the finger flexed by the pulley system; (b) in flexion the tendon moves anteriorly indicating a pulley injury.

Hand masses

- *Lipomas* are relatively common in the extremities. They are often fluctuant to palpation. On ultrasound they are the same echogenicity as fat. Small subcutaneous lipomas are almost always benign. If there is any doubt MRI can be used and benignity is assumed if the mass shows a uniform fatty appearance especially on sequences designed to eliminate signal from fat, e.g. STIR sequences (Fig. 5.23).

- *Fibromatosis* is well recognized in the palm and consists of nodular fibromas which are associated with dupuytrens contracture. The ultrasound appearance is variable and the fibromas are normally low signal on MRI. Digital fibromas are a rare infantile condition.

- *Ganglia* are common in the hands and are often attached to a tendon sheath. Diagnosis is usually made with ultrasound where they are normally well defined and fluid filled.

- *Haemangiomas* are common soft-tissue lesions especially in childhood. They are often associated with other conditions. They are classified according to the dominant vessel they contain. If the haemangioma contains calcification they can be seen on plain films. If not, ultrasound can normally detect vessels containing flow and the diagnosis can be confirmed by MRI.

- *Glomus tumours* are most common in a subungual position. They are tumours of the neuro-arterial glomus. They are often very painful and can cause well-defined bony erosion on plain film. They are hypoechoic on ultrasound and appear as low signal on T1 and high on T2 MRI sequences.

- *Giant cell tumours of the tendon sheath (GCT)* are histologically similar to pigmented villonodular synovitis (PVNS). They are associated with tendon sheaths. They are often hypoechoic on ultrasound and low signal on MRI due to the presence of haemosiderin. GCT's can appear similar to neurilemmomas, as a rule GCT's are more common distal to the metatarsophalangeal joints (Fig. 5.24).

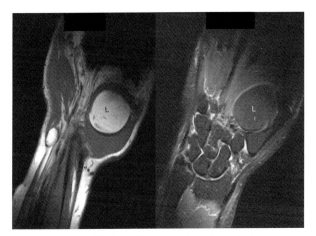

Fig. 5.23 T1 (left) and STIR (right) MRI of a large thenar lipoma (L). As the lipoma fully suppresses i.e. low signal on the STIR image malignancy is less likely.

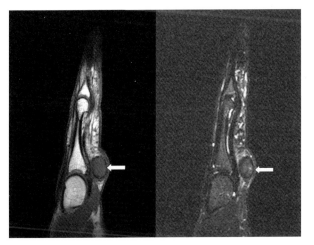

Fig. 5.24 T1 (left) and STIR (right) MRI show a low signal lesion intimately related to the flexor tendon. This is typical of a giant cell tumour.

Arthritis of the hands

Arthritis affecting the small joints of the hands represents a common manifestation of both degenerative and inflammatory joint diseases including rheumatoid arthritis, psoriatic arthritis, and crystal arthropathies. Recognition of specific joint pattern distribution may be helpful in establishing differential diagnoses of these joint diseases (Fig. 5.25).

Rheumatoid arthritis

The early changes on plain radiographs are soft-tissue swelling, juxta-articular osteoporosis, and joint space narrowing (Fig. 5.26).

In the later stage, chronic generalized osteoporosis, subchondral bone erosion especially radial-sided MCPJ, synovial cysts, subluxation, fibrous ankylosis or secondary OA in the small joints of the hands and the development of joint malalignment may occur (Fig. 5.27).

Features that distinguish RA from other inflammatory joint diseases include bilateral symmetrical involvement of the small joints of the hands sparing the DIP joints, juxta-articular osteopenia and lack of proliferative bone response.

Imaging modalities

Magnetic resonance imaging (MRI) and ultrasound (US)

MRI and US are more sensitive to inflammatory and destructive changes than conventional radiography and clinical examination. Early erosions, active synovitis and tenosynovitis are readily identified on both MRI and US.

The presence of intra-articular power Doppler signal may distinguish the hyperaemic response of active synovitis from inactive synovial thickening.

Psoriatic arthritis

Psoriatic arthritis often leads to a destructive arthropathy in the early stage of disease involving the DIP joints (Fig. 5.28). The PIP joints and MCP joints are commonly affected in an asymmetrical distribution.

The other characteristic radiological features that distinguish psoriatic arthritis from RA are:

- Soft-tissue swelling, often with a sausage-digit appearance (dactylitis)
- Lower frequency of periarticular osteopaenia
- Marginal erosions with adjacent proliferation of bone resulting in 'whiskering'
- Irregular shaft periostitis
- Osteolysis with pencil-in-cup deformity and acro-osteolysis
- A tendency to ankylosis of the joint
- Enthesopathy

Imaging modalities

Magnetic resonance imaging (MRI) and ultrasound (US)

These extrasynovial abnormalities of enthesopathy and soft-tissue inflammation are more readily demonstrable on US and MRI than conventional radiographs. On MRI, dactylitis appears as tenosynovitis and effusion, sometimes associated with small joint synovitis.

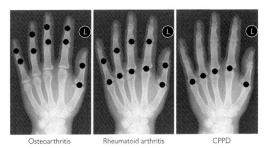

Osteoarthritis   Rheumatoid arthritis   CPPD

Fig. 5.25 Typical joint distribution of arthritis in the hands.

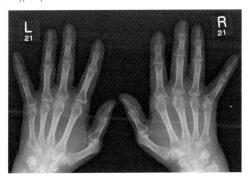

Fig. 5.26 Rheumatoid arthritis. Marked joint space narrowing with adjacent osteopaenia are demonstrated over the MCP joints with relative sparing of the more distal joints.

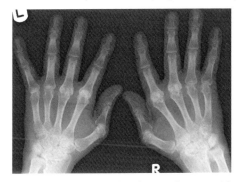

Fig. 5.27 Bilateral symmetrical arthropathy with erosive changes over left and right index, middle and little MCP and right ring MCP joints are demonstrated here. There is associated ulnar deviation over the right MCP joints with erosive changes over carpal bones and radioulnar joints bilaterally. Secondary degenerative changes are seen over carpal bones bilaterally.

Crystal arthropathies

There are three types of crystal which produce disease: monosodium urate, calcium pyrophosphate dehydrate (CPPD), and calcium hydroxyapetite.

Clinical features

The crystals in CPPD may deposit in the synovium, periarticular tissues, hyaline and fibrocartilage (chondrocalcinosis). Within the hand, the MCP joints are frequently affected, most commonly the second and third MCP joints. Secondary causes for CCPD such as haemachromatosis should be excluded in a subset of patients (Fig. 5.29).

The radiological appearance of CPPD arthropathy is variable with beak-like projections from index and middle metacarpal heads, and features of degenerative joint disease with cartilage loss, sclerosis, and subchondral cyst formation. Typically there is absence of erosive disease.

Similarly, hydroxyapetite deposition disease has a predilection for the MCP joints.

Often the crystals are not visible radiologically. However, crystals may also result in calcification that appears as amorphous or cloudlike areas. This may lead to a severely destructive arthropathy which resembles osteoarthritis, with joint space narrowing, subchondral sclerosis, osseous debris, and joint disorganization.

Imaging modalities

Radiography

Plain radiographs of urate arthropathy or gout will demonstrate soft-tissue opacifications with densities between soft tissue and bone, characteristic punched-out defect with a thin sclerotic margin and overhanging edges secondary to periosteal new bone apposition, and osteophytes at the margins of opacifications or erosions.

Ultrasound (US)

US may be more sensitive and may reveal bright stippled foci with hyper-echoic soft-tissue areas. Presence of power Doppler signals may identify actively inflamed joints.

Magnetic resonance imaging (MRI)

US, CT and MRI may detect subclinical tophi. On MRI, these appear as inter-mediate or low-signal masses on both T1- and T2-weighted sequences.

Osteoarthritis

Distinguishing features of OA include subchondral sclerosis, seen as increased bone density around the joints, osteophytes, subchondral cysts, and loose bone fragments within the joints typically in the later stages of disease.

Clinically, presence of Bouchard's and Heberden's nodes over the posterolateral aspects of the PIP and DIP joints respectively are consistent with nodular generalized osteoarthritis. The first carpometacarpal, MCP and interphalangeal joints of the thumb are also commonly affected. The index and middle MCP joints may be affected in some cases.

Loss of cortical integrity over the surface of the joint in severe cases may be labelled as erosive OA. Compared to RA, the erosive changes are central rather than marginal and may heal leaving a gull-wing appearance with ankylosis of the IP joints (Fig. 5.30).

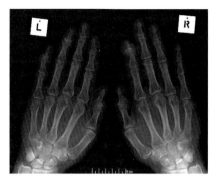

Fig. 5.28 Psoriatic arthritis. Asymmetrical destructive erosions demonstrated over distal joints of right index, left ring and little fingers.

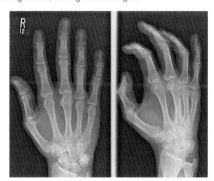

Fig. 5.29 Hooked osteophytes of the index and middle MCP joints of haemochromatosis.

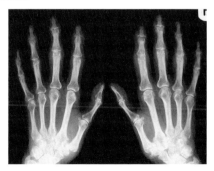

Fig. 5.30 Osteoarthritis. Osteophytes, as seen here over the DIP and PIP joints, are the *sine qua non* of osteoarthritis resulting in a gull-wing appearance.

Investigating elbow problems

Anatomy

The elbow joint (Fig. 6.1) is a hinge joint that also allows the forearm to supinate and pronate. The humerus articulates with the ulna at the trochlea. The large trochlear groove in the ulna and the coronoid process constitute the hinge joint of the elbow. The radius rotates on the capitellum of the humerus and the ulna. The radioulnar joint at the elbow is formed by the annular ligament and the radial notch of the ulna. There are depressions in the distal humerus, the largest of which are the olecranon fossa and the coronoid fossa, that accommodate the olecranon and coronoid processes in full flexion and extension.

The appearance of the ossification centres in children is the key to understanding fractures in the immature skeleton (Fig. 6.2). They appear in a set order:

* **C**apitellum   1 yr
* **R**adial head   5 yrs
* **I**nternal (medial) epicondyle   6yrs
* **T**rochlea   9yrs
* **O**lecranon   10yrs
* **L**ateral epicondyle   11yrs

The dates of appearance are approximate but the order remains the same.

The key injury that requires the CRITOL sequence for diagnosis is that the internal epicondyle must appear before the trochlea. If the trochlea is seen first, a displaced medial epicondyle should be considered.

The medial and lateral epicondyles are the origins of the common flexor and extensor origins respectively. Pain at these sites can be due to tennis and golfers elbow (☐ Tennis and golfer's elbow, p.188).

The biceps tendon inserts into the radial tubercle which is unusually the site of a biceps rupture or bursitis.

The main neurovascular structures pass the elbow in the antecubital fossa, apart from the ulnar nerve which passes behind the medial epicondyle in the cubital tunnel.

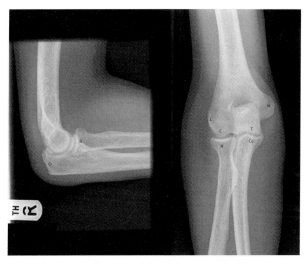

Fig. 6.1 Elbow anatomy. R, radial head; C, capitellum; T, trochlea; Co, coronoid; L, lateral epicondyle; M, medial epicondyle.

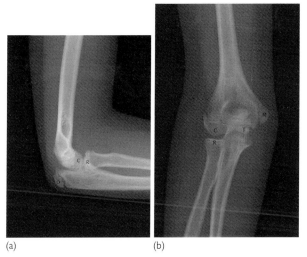

(a)   (b)

Fig 6.2 (a) AP and (b) lateral image of a normal child's elbow showing the ossification centres.

Fractures

The presence of the anterior and posterior fat pad signs can be helpful in diagnosing fractures. This is more reliable in the mature skeleton.

Children

Due to the age of appearance of the ossification centres in children fractures can be easy to miss. Dislocation is more common than in the mature skeleton. A systematic approach is essential.

- First, the anterior humeral line should be traced and it should normally intersect with the middle third of the capitellum. If it does not a supracondylar fracture should be suspected (Fig. 6.3).
- Then the radio–capitellum line should be traced to check for radial head dislocation.
- Fractures of the condyles can cause confusion. The normal appearance of the condyles can be variable and should be looked up in anatomical and normal variation reference books. The lateral condyle is more commonly injured and is usually seen as a widened gap between the condyle and the humerus.
- If there is a trochlear ossification centre without a medial epicondyle, the medial epicondyle may have been pulled into the joint. The key to this diagnosis is CRITOL. The medial epicondyle always appears before the trochlear.

Adults

In the mature skeleton the most reliable sign of acute effusion is elevation of the fat pads, especially the posterior (Fig. 6.4). If both are elevated but no obvious fracture is visible, a non-displaced radial head fracture is the most likely injury. Effusions are not diagnostic however. Radial neck fractures can be extra-capsular so may not result in an effusion.

The Monteggia fracture is a combination of a radial head dislocation and an ulnar fracture.

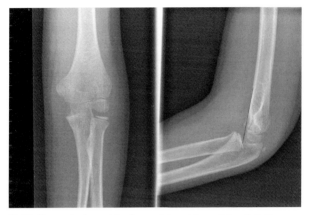

Fig 6.3 The anterior humeral line does not intersect the capitellum, indicating a supracondylar fracture.

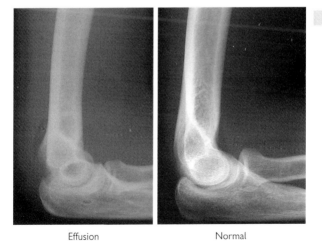

Effusion   Normal

Fig 6.4 The elevated anterior fat pad and posterior fat pad are obvious when compared to a normal elbow.

Intra-articular loose bodies

The most common cause for loose bodies in the elbow joint is trauma. Degeneration is the next most common cause.

The bodies are made up of cartilage alone, cartilage and bone or just bone.

These bodies can cause locking, pain, and restriction of movement. A common place for them to collect is the olecranon fossa.

Imaging modalities

- Imaging can be problematic. Larger loose bodies can be seen on plain film but smaller ones may not be seen. Occasionally degenerative change may cause so much calcification that plain film cannot determine if a body is in the joint.
- MR and MR arthrography are not 100% reliable as the signal characteristics of the loose body can make it difficult to see. Small bony loose bodies are proton-dense and may be difficult to detect (Fig. 6.5). Non-arthrographic MR has better exclusion value when there is joint effusion present,
- In the presence of an effusion some intra-articular loose bodies can be seen using ultrasound. Conventional and CT arthrography can be more reliable than MR.
- Imaging can determine if loose bodies are present and the location to guide surgical planning but they may have moved before any operative intervention.

Synovial osteochondromatosis

- This condition, caused by synovial hypertrophy and calcification, can result in multiple loose bodies.
- If these loose bodies are calcified then they can be seen on plain film as multiple dense nodules within the joint capsule.
- If they have not calcified then MR can show the nodules as low signal on T2-weighted images within the high-signal synovium.
- Treatment is by surgical excision of the synovium.

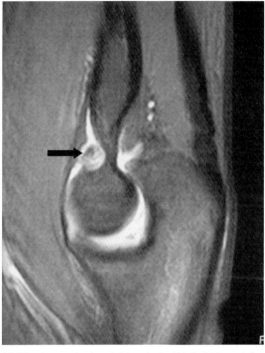

Fig. 6.5 MR arthrogram showing a dark loose body within the joint capsule (arrow).

Osteochondral injury (osteochondritis dissecans)

The capitellum is the usual site for osteochondritis dissecans of the elbow. It is more common in adolescents than adults and is associated with throwing activities. The aetiology is probably a combination of repeated valgus force on the elbow and an immature cartilaginous surface. Osteochondritis dissecans of the elbow in the skeletally immature is part of the 'Little League Elbow Syndrome'.

Clinical features

The symptoms are pain that worsens with activity and limited movements. Patients sometimes report a clicking sensation.

Osteochondritis dissecans is divided into Type I, no fracture or displacement; Type II, evidence of cartilagenous fracture or minimal displacement; and Type III, completely displaced with a loose body.

Plain films are normally highly suggestive with CT and MR normally characterizing the extent of the lesion and looking for intra-articular loose bodies (Fig. 6.6).

A differential is osteochondrosis of the capitellum (Panner's disease). This appears as a fragmented capitellar epiphysis and even avascular necrosis. Panner's disease is more common in pre-teenage males and osteochondtritis dissecans in post-teen males. Panner's disease classically does not progress.

Elbow pain in children is one of the situations where a comparison film of the asymptomatic side may be of benefit.

Treatment of osteochodritis dissecans is normally conservative for Type 1 with surgery for more severe cases to remove loose bodies or k-wire the osteochondral defect.

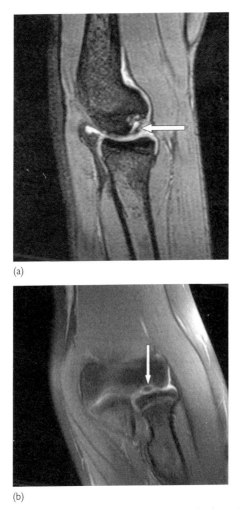

(a)

(b)

Fig. 6.6 Sagittal (a) and coronal (b) MRI of an osteochondral defect (arrows).

Ulnar collateral ligament injury of the elbow

The ulnar collateral ligament (UCL) of the elbow comprises three bands: anterior, posterior and transverse ligaments. The anterior band provides the major contribution to valgus stability.

Repetitive throwing motions and traumatic valgus stress to the elbow in association with acute elbow dislocation are important causes of UCL injury. During the acceleration phase of the overhead throw, the forearm lags behind the upper arm and generates valgus stress. This force may overcome the tensile strength of the UCL and cause microscopic tears or acute rupture.

Discomfort over the medial elbow may occur during the acceleration phase of the overhead throw. The pain may become chronic or recurrent with frequent throwing activities, and may be associated with a popping sensation. Localized tenderness and swelling may be detected approximately 2cm distal to the medial epicondyle. Loss of elbow range of motion may be evident. Pain may be reproduced on making a clenched fist and valgus stress with elbow in 25° in flexion.

Imaging modalities

Radiology

Plain radiography may reveal an avulsion fragment and ossification of UCL. A bone spur may form at the ulnar insertion. Plain radiographs will also rule out other causes of elbow pain such as epicondylar fractures or posterior olecranon loose bodies.

Magnetic resonance imaging (MRI)

MRI (Fig. 6.7) is useful to detect UCL rupture. Partial tears can be difficult to diagnose. Discontinuity of the UCL provides direct evidence of rupture with loss of distinction or laxity of the ligament. Increased signal intensity in the UCL and adjacent tissues on T1- and T2-weighted images suggests haemorrhage and oedema associated with the injury.

Ultrasound (US)

Dynamic US may be helpful in evaluation of ligamentous laxity in throwing athletes.

Initial conservative management with rest, physiotherapy, non-steroidal anti-inflammatory drugs and steroid injections of UCL injury is often tried but primary reconstructive repair of the UCL with tendon graft may be necessary.

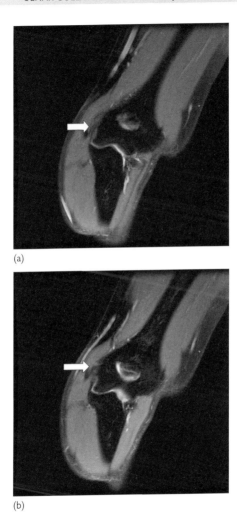

(a)

(b)

Fig. 6.7 UCL injury. MRI with full elbow extension (coronal view, T2-weighted image) reveals increase in signal with discontinuity of the UCL.

Tennis and golfer's elbow

These will present as pain around the elbow joint. Both conditions may be diagnosed on history and clinical examination. These two conditions may occasionally coexist but in general bilateral elbow pain or pain with tenderness at more than one site suggests another condition. The localized nature of these conditions helps to distinguish them from elbow pain arising from arthritis of the joint itself or referred pain from the wrist or cervical spine.

Lateral epicondylitis
Clinical features
Lateral epicondylitis or tennis elbow presents with variable pain, from mild aching on using the arm to severe pain affecting sleep. The pain is provoked by gripping and twisting movements. Tenderness of the epicondyle is noticed by the patient on knocking their elbow. The pain may radiate down the posterolateral aspect of the forearm.

Paraesthesia over the arm is unusual and may suggest neural compression.

Clinical examination
The elbow joint is normal and moves freely without any inflammatory swelling. The pain is reproduced with resisted extension of the wrist and forced radial deviation of the wrist with the elbow held in the extended position.

Imaging modalities
Radiography
Plain radiographs may detect irregular calcification of the lateral epicondyle in chronic cases.

Ultrasound (US)
US may reveal thickening of the tendon with reduced echogenicity (Fig. 6.9) and increased blood flow on doppler.

Magnetic resonance imaging (MRI)
MRI may demonstrate focal increased signal intensity of the extensor tendons adjacent to their insertion on the lateral epicondyle.

Management is primarily conservative, with rest, anti-inflammatory medication and local injection therapy. Chronic cases may be treated with surgical release of the extensor tendon.

Medial epicondylitis
This relates to overuse injury of the common tendinous origin of the flexor–pronator muscles as a result of repetitive activity. It is commonly observed among manual workers, throwing sports and in golfers, hence the term golfer's elbow.

Clinical features
Patients complain of aching sensation over the medial elbow and proximal flexor compartment of the forearm. There may be pain resulting in reduction in range of motion in particular on full extension. Tenderness is localized over the medial epicondyle. Resisted wrist flexion with the elbow flexed and forearm supinated reproduces the pain.

Imaging modalities
Ultrasound (US)
US will detect similar abnormalities to those noted in lateral epicondylitis.

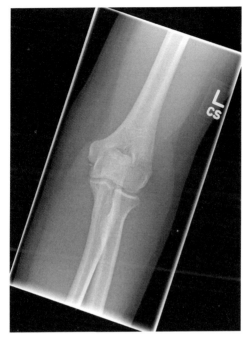

Fig. 6.8 Plain radiograph of elbow reveal enthesopathy at the lateral epicondyle.

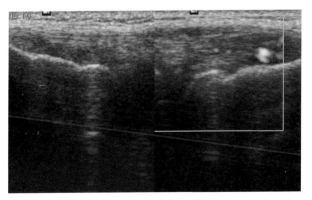

Fig. 6.9 US of affected area demonstrates thickening of the extensor tendon with increase in Doppler flow signal (right hand image) consistent with localized inflammation. A normal extensor tendon origin is shown on the left for comparison.

Arthritis of the elbow

The elbow is a common site for arthritis which can be due to infection, trauma, degenerative osteoarthritis, and inflammatory arthritis (crystal arthropathy and rheumatoid arthritis).

Septic arthritis and crystal arthropathy

Both may present in similar manner with acute pain, swelling and erythema. Previous history of gout or pseudogout attacks, presence of gouty tophi, involvement of the first metatarsophalangeal joint, presence of risk factors such as diuretic therapy, alcohol abuse, or renal insufficiency may suggest crystal-induced arthritis.

Both conditions may coexist and analysis of synovial fluid for Gram stain, crystals and cultures are paramount for precise diagnosis.

Osteoarthritis of the elbow

Primary elbow osteoarthritis typically affects middle-aged men who perform manual labour and presents as impingement pain with loss of terminal extension of the elbow. Loose bodies, osteophytes, and capsular contracture are frequently found. Painful catching or locking may represent the presence of loose or synovialized osteocartilaginous fragments.

Plain film radiographs characteristically demonstrate ulnotrochlear joint space narrowing with anterior and medial osteophyte involving the coronoid process with posteromedial osteophyte on the olecranon process. Corresponding osteophytes on the humeral side are found in the coronoid and olecranon fossae. Radiocapitellar and proximal radioulnar involvement may be seen in advanced stages of disease (Fig. 6.10).

Rheumatoid arthritis

Elbow synovitis is present in half or more of the patients. Pain occurs throughout the arc of motion associated with loss of extension and forearm rotation. Active synovitis is readily palpated at the site of the groove between the olecranon and the lateral epicondyle. Bulging tenderness and flexion contracture are typical findings. Nodules may be found over the olecranon bursa and proximal extensor surface of the ulna.

Compression of the ulnar nerve posteromedially to the elbow may result in paraesthesias in the fourth and fifth fingers.

Radiological features typical for RA include symmetrical joint space narrowing, periarticular erosions and disuse osteopenia. Marked articular destruction with extensive loss of subchondral bone may occur in severe cases (Fig. 6.11).

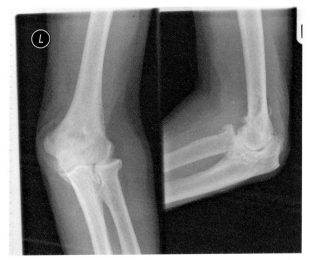

Fig. 6.10 Osteoarthritis: anteroposterior radiograph reveals loss of definition of the coronoid and olecranon fossae due to thickening of the bone in this region and osteophyte formation. Lateral radiograph demonstrates the osteophytes on the olecranon. The anterior osteophytes are sometimes more difficult to distinguish.

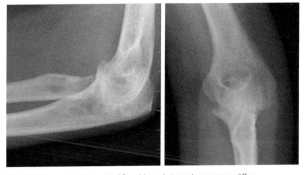

Fig. 6.11 Rheumatoid arthritis: AP and lateral views demonstrate diffuse involvement of joint with marked joint space narrowing and extensive erosion in olecranon articulation with trochlea of the humerus seeming to 'dig into' the olecranon.

Triceps tendinitis

Repetitive forced extension of the elbow can result in tendinopathy of the triceps tendon as it inserts into the olecranon. This is more common in adult throwing athletes such as javelin throwers.

- The patients suffer posterior elbow pain on extension which is often chronic.
- This condition can be divided into patients with and without an olecranon bony spur.
- Plain films can show the olecranon spur and ultrasound can show the triceps tendinopathy.
- Treatment is conservative with rest, non-steroidal anti-inflammatories (NSAIDs) and time. Surgical management is more common in patients with a spur which can be removed and the tendon repaired.

Tendon rupture around the elbow

The two tendons most likely to rupture around the elbow are the biceps and triceps.

Distal biceps rupture is uncommon and is usually caused by excessive tension while in a fixed flexion position. A popping sensation is often felt. The lacertus fibrosus aponeurosis inserts into the deep fascia of the forearm. If both the tendon and the aponeurosis rupture it is usually clinically obvious with a palpable defect and retracted tendon. If the aponeurosis is intact it prevents retraction of the torn tendon making clinical assessment problematic.

Imaging modalities

Ultrasound (US)

Ultrasound can usually see a defect and the retracted tendon. However, the twisting distal course of the tendon and an artefact called anisotropy commonly seen in tendons can make diagnosis difficult.

Magnetic resonance imaging (MRI)

MRI can be used in these cases.

Treatment of biceps rupture has been controversial between conservative and surgical re-implantation. Recent studies have shown surgical treatment to offer a better outcome.

Triceps rupture is less common, the usual pattern is a fracture of the olecranon after a fall. Triceps rupture is usually obvious clinically and ultrasound can diagnose the injury.

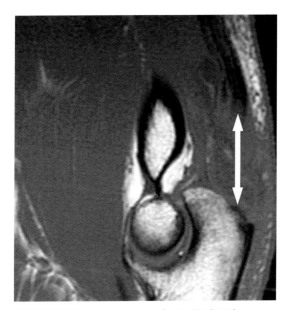

Fig. 6.12 Sagittal MRI shows a torn triceps tendon insertion (arrow).

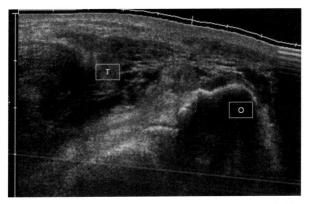

Fig. 6.13 Panoramic ultrasound clearly shows the olecranon (O) and the end of the detached triceps tendon (T).

Biceps bursitis and rupture

Biceps rupture

The biceps brachii muscle is one of the main flexors and supinators of the elbow. Avulsion of the distal radial attachment of biceps usually occurs in men over 50 years following forced flexion against strong resistance.

Patients will experience an acute tearing sensation with a snap. The tendon is usually not palpable having retracted into the forearm.

This may be demonstrated with dynamic US or MRI (Fig. 6.14) with discontinuity and retraction of the tendon, often with intervening haematoma. Most tears occur 1–2cm above the radial tuberosity, where there is poor vascular supply.

The treatment of choice for complete rupture of the distal biceps tendon is early surgical repair. Partial tears are often treated conservatively with local or systemic analgesics.

Biceps bursitis

Numerous bursae are present around the elbow. The bicipitoradial bursa lies between the distal biceps tendon and the anterior part of the radial tuberosity. As the forearm is pronated, the radial tuberosity rotates from a medial to a posterior position. The biceps tendon curves around the radius, compressing the interposed bursa.

Repetitive mechanical trauma is the most frequent cause of bicipitoradial bursitis: other causes include infection, inflammatory arthropathy, chemical synovitis, bone proliferation, pigmented villonodular synovitis, and synovial chondromatosis

When inflamed, the bursa may enlarge with a palpable mass in the cubital fossa and it may cause compression of the adjacent median or posterior interosseous nerves.

Treatment is largely conservative with local aspiration and corticosteroid injection.

Imaging modalities

Ultrasound (US)

Ultrasound may show a fusiform anechoic or hypoechoic lesion (Fig. 6.15).

Magnetic resonance imaging (MRI)

MRI imaging will demonstrate fluid distension of the bursa with hypointensity on T1-weighted images and hyperintensity on T2-weighted images. MRI will also distinguish bursitis from other condtions including synovial chondromatosis, pigmented villonodular synovitis, tenosynovitis, and ganglion cyst.

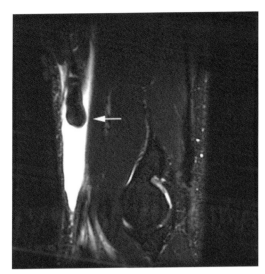

Fig. 6.14 MRI on T2-weighted images (sagittal view) demonstrates (arrow) retraction of the biceps tendon with discontinuity of the tendon.

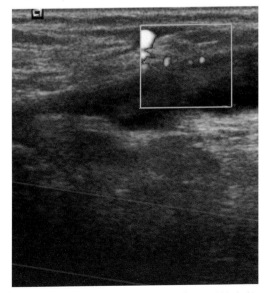

Fig. 6.15 US of the elbow demonstrates inflammatory changes within the biceps bursa.

Ulnar neuropathy

At the level of the elbow, the ulnar nerve is normally located between the olecranon process and the medial epicondyle. Lesions in the ulnar retro-epicondylar groove account for most cases of neural compression. The nerve follows a constrained path and movement of the elbow therefore requires the nerve to both stretch and slide through the cubital tunnel. Subluxation of the ulnar nerve may occur as it is slides out of the cubital tunnel and over the medial epicondyle during elbow flexion.

Other risk factors for ulnar nerve entrapment include:

- Diabetes
- Occupation-related activities with frequent elbow flexion
- Fractures with valgus deformity
- Recurrent dislocation
- Pressure over ulnar groove

Clinical features

Initially, most patients may complain of intermittent numbness and tingling over the little and ring fingers. Pain is not a prominent feature, and loss of motor function is usually the dominant clinical problem. Percussion on the nerve and sustained elbow flexion with the wrist extended may reproduce the symptoms.

Most patients will recover spontaneously or with conservative treatment with avoidance of elbow trauma or excessive movement and the appropriate use of elbow pads. Surgery is reserved for difficult cases.

Imaging modalities

Radiography

Radiographs are performed to identify any bony or joint abnormalities. The diagnostic yield of nerve conduction studies for ulnar nerve neuropathy is less than that for carpal tunnel syndrome and the interpretation of the data is often difficult.

Ultrasound (US)

US in flexion and extension may demonstrate dynamic nerve impingement. With ulnar nerve dislocation, the abrupt displacement of the nerve medial to the medial epicondyle produces a snapping sensation felt through the transducer. Displacement may be asymptomatic. US may also reveal a fusiform hypoechoic swelling of the ulnar nerve with loss of the fascicular pattern The cross-sectional area of the compressed nerve is greater than that of the corresponding nerves in the opposite normal arm.

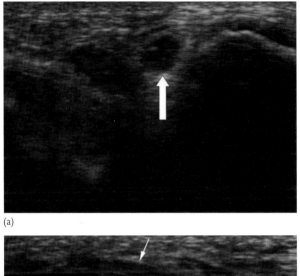

(a)

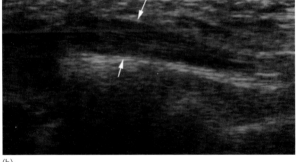

(b)

Fig. 6.16 Transverse (a) and longitudinal (b) ultrasound of a normal ulnar nerve at the elbow.

Investigating foot and ankle problems

Anatomy

Functionally it can be helpful to think of the ankle, hindfoot, midfoot, and forefoot as separate entities.

- The ankle comprises the distal ends of the tibia and fibula which articulate with the trochlear surface of the talus to form a synovial hinge joint constrained medially and laterally by the malleoli (Fig. 7.1).
- The mortice-type structure is stable under load although the talus is narrower posteriorly (Fig. 7.2 black arrowheads) and the ankle joint is less stable in plantarflexion.
- Integrity between the tibia and fibula at the distal end is maintained by the interosseous membrane and the tibiofibular ligament.

The ankle is surrounded by ligamentous structures (Figs 7.3 and 7.4 white arrows):

- The large, fan-shaped deltoid ligament on the medial side
- Three lateral ligaments—the anterior talofibular (Fig. 7.4 white arrow) the calcaneofibular and the posterior talofibular on the lateral side (Fig. 7.3 white arrowheads).
- Deep to these lie the posterior and lateral talocalcaneal ligaments.
- Anterior stability is provided by an anterior (tibiotalar) ligament.

Tendons passing around the ankle are constrained within a series of extensor and flexor retinaculae. For several centimetres proximal and distal to this region, the tendons are invested in a synovial sheath which should be considered when investigating tenosynovitis.

The tendons pass, along with a neurovascular bundle, in three compartments; the anterior, the posteromedial and the posterolateral. Several mnemonics have been developed to help memorize the sequences and these can be particularly helpful for interpreting anatomy (Fig. 7.4).

- For the anterior compartment—Tom Hates Dick.
  - Medial to lateral Tibialis anterior (Ta), extensor Hallucis longus (He) and extensor Digitorum longus (De). (Note also the saphenous vein.)
- Posteromedial compartment—Tom, Dick and (A Very Nervous) Harry (arrows Fig. 7.2)
  - From medial malleolus to tendo Achilles: Tibialis posterior (T), flexor Digitorum longus (D), (posterior tibial Artery, tibial Vein, tibial Nerve) flexor Hallucis longus (H).
- The posterolateral compartment contains the peroneus longus (PL) and peroneus brevis (PB) tendons as well as the sural nerve.

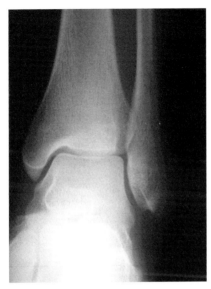

Fig. 7.1 Anterior posterior (AP) view plain radiograph of the normal ankle.

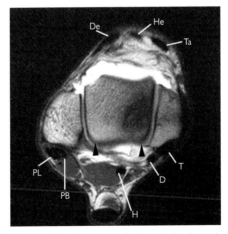

Fig. 7.2 T1 transverse MRI of the normal ankle demonstrating the tendons Tibialis anterior (Ta), extensor Hallucis longus (He), extensor Digitorum longus (De), Tibialis posterior (T), flexor Digitorum longus (D), and flexor Hallucis longus (H).

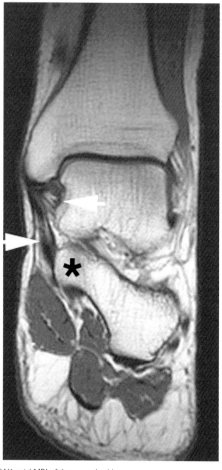

Fig. 7.3 TW1 axial MRI of the normal ankle.

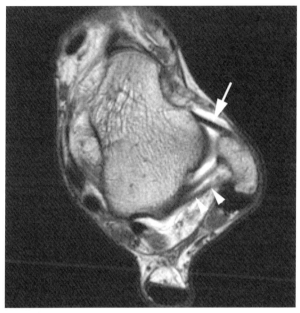

Fig. 7.4 TW1 transverse MRI of the normal ankle clearly demonstrating ligaments.

The tendo Achilles lies some distance from the ankle posteriorly and crosses both the ankle and subtalar joints.

- The tendo Achilles send slips around the posterior calcaneus and is partly contiguous with the plantar fascia (Fig. 7.5 white arrowhead).
- The Achilles is not invested in a synovial sheath although the retrocalcaneal bursa, which lies between the distal end of the tendon and the superior upper third of the posterior calcaneus (Fig. 7.5 white arrow), does have synovial lining.

The subtalar joint is a complex three-facet joint responsible for inversion/eversion and pronation/supination of the foot.

- The talus sits on calcaneus on the superior surface of the sustentaculum tali which provides stability and a point of routing for the posteromedial soft tissues (Fig. 7.3 asterisk).
- Anteriorly there is a space between the talus and the calcaneus, increased on plantarflexion and inversion—the sinus tarsi (Fig. 7.6 black arrowhead).
- The talus receives no muscular insertions and so subtalar motions are passive. For this reason the ankle and subtalar joint can often be considered functionally as a single unit.

The midfoot region is bounded proximally by the talonavicular and calcaneocuboid joints (known collectively as the midtarsal joint) (Fig. 7.5 white acute arrowhead) and distally by the tarsometatarsal joints (known collectively as Lisfranc's joint) (Fig. 7.5 white acute arrowhead).

This region is important to the stability of the medial arch of the foot during function and so is supported by many ligamentous structures, intrinsic musculature and a thick, fibrous band, the plantar aponeurosis or plantar fascia.

The talonavicular joint is essentially a ball and socket joint although it is complex in make-up comprising:

- the talus and navicular
- an articulation with a small portion of the calcaneus
- and unusually a fibrocartilaginous articulation with a dense plantar calcaneonavicular ligament known as the 'spring ligament'.
- A further ligament from the calcaneus to the navicular, the bifurcate ligament, also enhances mid-tarsal stability. This mechanism can be compromised in inflammatory disease.
- The navicular articulates distally with three small cuneiform bones, which in turn articulate with the medial three metatarsals forming part of Lisfranc's joint (Fig. 7.7 black arrowheads). There many articulations between the small bones of the tarsus.
- The tendon of tibialis posterior passes behind the medial malleolus and inserts into the tuberosity of the navicular and other tarsal bones.

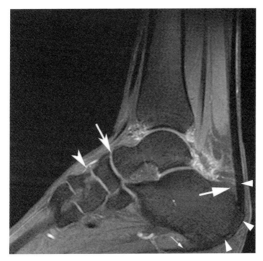

Fig. 7.5 TW1 post-gadolinium sagittal MRI of the normal ankle.

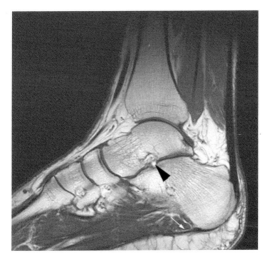

Fig. 7.6 TW1 sagittal MRI of the normal ankle.

On the lateral side of the foot:
- The calcaneocuboid joint (Fig. 7.7 white arrow) provides small amounts of motion, mainly dorsi- and plantarflexion.
- The peroneal tendons (peroneus longus and peroneus brevis) pass behind the lateral malleolus (Fig. 7.2) with peroneus brevis inserting directly into the base of the 5th metatarsal
- Peroneus longus passes via the cuboid notch across the plantar surface of the foot inserting into the base of the first metatarsal.
- Anteriorly the tendon of extensor digitorum longus divides into four slips and pass along the metatarsals.
- The distal aspect of the cuboid articulates directly with the 4th and 5th metatarsal (Fig. 7.7 short white arrows) to form the lateral part of Lisfranc's joint.

Distal to Lisfranc's joint is the forefoot, comprising:
- the five metatarsals
- their associated metatarsophalangeal (MTP) joints, and the phalanges and their associated joints.

The five metatarsals are weight-bearing structures loaded at the proximal and distal ends. The first metatarsal is considerably greater in diameter than the lesser metatarsals, highlighting the importance of the medial column to normal function. Stress reactions/fractures can occur in the thin neck region of the metatarsal bones.

Distally the synovial MTP joints form a smooth arc across the forefoot.
- The five MTP joints are bound together by a deep transverse metatarsal ligament.
- Individually, joint integrity is maintained by a capsule, two collateral ligaments and a plantar ligament containing a fibrocartilaginous plate.
- The first MTP joint has a broad, longitudinally grooved inferior surface and two sesamoid bones (Fig. 7.8 white asterisks) provide insertions for the medial and lateral heads of flexor hallucis brevis under the joint.

The neurovascular bundles supplying the toes pass close to the MTP joints and may be involved in pathology. Resulting disorders such as intermetatarsal bursitis and Morton's neuroma are covered later in this chapter.

Finally the digits themselves comprise multiple small segments.
- The hallux comprises only two phalanges while the lesser toes generally comprise three.
- The synovial joints are all stabilized by medial and lateral collateral ligaments as well as thickened plantar ligaments.
- Many tendons insert in this region and so insertions and entheseal structures abound.
- The extensor tendons insert into all three phalanges superiorly.
- Inferiorly the interossei insert into the proximal phalanx and the long flexors into the distal phalanx.

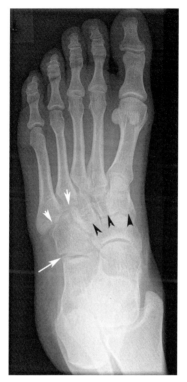

Fig. 7.7 Plain film radiograph demonstrating normal forefoot anatomy.

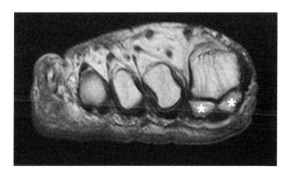

Fig. 7.8 Axial MRI demonstrating normal forefoot anatomy.

Ankle osteoarthritis

- Osteoarthritis (OA) is not commonly seen in the ankle (Figs 7.9, 7.10)
- Ankle OA is usually the result of major trauma (e.g. complex ankle fracture), repeated minor trauma (e.g. recurrent ankle sprains) or following inflammatory arthritis
- May be osteoarthritis elsewhere (such as hallux abductovalgus and Heberden nodes) so that this is part of generalized osteoarthritis but site-specific because of injury
- Main clinical features are pain, particularly on weight-bearing, swelling, limitation of movement and difficulty walking
- Swelling most often due to new bone at joint margins (osteophytes) but can also be due to low grade synovitis

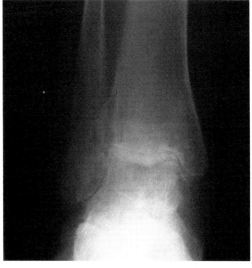

Fig. 7.9 Plain, antero-posterior view radiograph showing asteoarthritis of the ankle (tibio-talar) joint. Note uniform joint space narrowing, osteophytes, sub-chondral cysts and sub-chondral sclerosis.

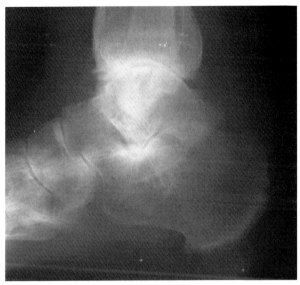

Fig. 7.10 Plain lateral radiograph of osteoarthritis of the ankle (tibio-talar) joint. Note again the uniform joint space narrowing, osteophytes, sub-chondral cysts and sub-chondral sclerosis.

Ankle inflammatory arthritis

The ankle joint complex consists of tibiotalar, subtalar, talonavicular and calcaneocuboid joints). In terms of frequency in the clinic caused by:
- Rheumatoid arthritis
- Psoriatic arthritis
- Reactive arthritis and other spondyloarthropathies
- Miscellaneous conditions such as sarcoidosis and pigmented villonodular synovitis (PVNS)

Major clinical signs are soft-tissue swelling (along the anterior line of the tibiotalar joint, at either side of the Achilles just proximal to the insertion, and the sinus tarsi) and deformity (pes planovalgus, although ankle varus occasionally encountered).

Rheumatoid arthritis (Figs 7.11a and 7.11b)
- Ankle joint complex less commonly involved compared to forefoot joints—about 40% after 10 years
- Frequency of joint involvement: talonavicular > subtalar > tibiotalar but all can be involved and communication between joints occurs
- Extra-articular features:
  - soft-tissue structures (tibialis posterior tendon, peroneal tendons and deltoid ligament of the ankle) affected and probably play a major part in joint deformity
  - rheumatoid nodules in Achilles tendon or heel
  - rheumatoid vasculitis as nail fold infarcts or leg ulcers
- Most common deformity is ankle valgus at the subtalar joint with forefoot pronation, loss of longitudinal arch and inferior displacement of navicular bone

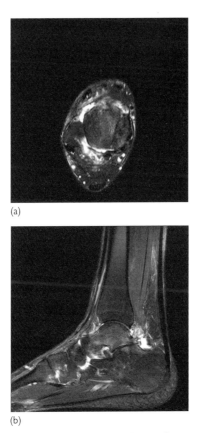

(a)

(b)

Fig. 7.11 (a) and (b) T2W MRI scans of the ankle showing inflammation due to rheumatoid arthritis. High signal on these images indicate joint effusion and synovitis. There is also abnormal signal in the bone due to bone oedema.

Psoriatic arthritis

- May present with isolated inflammation of the ankle joint complex
- Associated features include:
  - frequent enthesitis at the Achilles insertion (Fig. 7.12a) and the plantar fascia insertion on the calcaneum at the medial tubercle (Fig. 7.12b)
  - Dactylitis of a toe or finger
  - Nail changes of psoriasis

Reactive arthritis and other spondyloarthropathies

- Lower limb large-joint inflammatory arthritis common presentation in reactive arthritis
- May be associated conjunctivitis, urethritis, and diarrhoea
- Dactylitis and psoriaform skin lesions (keratoderma blennorhagica) may also be seen

Miscellaneous conditions such as sarcoidosis and PVNS

- Ankle inflammation seen in sarcoidosis in association with juxta-articular erythema nodosum and, although severe, is usually self-limiting in a matter of days
- PVNS affects isolated joints, usually the knee but can be seen in any synovial structure, including the major tendon sheaths around the ankle

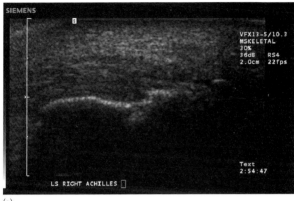

(a)

Fig. 7.12 (a) Longitudinal ultrasound scan of the Achilles tendon showing thickening and irregularity at the point of insertion, due to erosions.

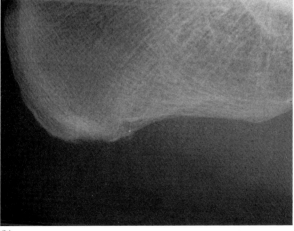

(b)

Fig. 7.12 (b) Lateral radiograph of calcaneus demonstrating cortical erosions at the point of insertion of the plantar fascia.

Osteochondral injuries

- Inversion sprains around the ankle are common both in and out of sport
- Most sprains are minor but the severest can result in ligamentous rupture and osteochondral defects in the articular surface of the talus and the tibia
- The most important risk factor for sprain is a previous sprain so adequate treatment of a first sprain is very important
- Most sprains present at A&E and undergo X-ray investigation. Often, they also receive inappropriate advice on early management (📖 Ankle fractures, p.224). Investigations are rarely of help initially.
- The more severe sprains are associated with ligament rupture, avulsion injury (at the base of the 5th metatarsal) and osteochondral injuries (Fig 7.13a, b, c). For sprained ankles that do not recover these factors should be considered. In these cases imaging diagnostics are required and, in some cases, a surgical solution is necessary.

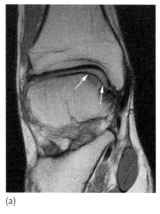

(a)

Fig. 7.13 (a) Coronal Proton Density weighted PDw MRI showing medial cartilage defect (arrow).

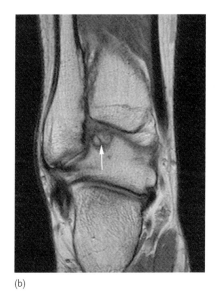

(b)

Fig. 7.13 (b) Coronal PD w MRI showing posterolateral cartilage defect and subchondrial cystic change (arrow).

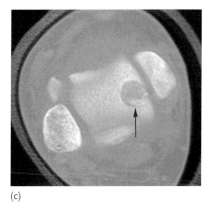

(c)

Fig. 7.13 (c) Axial CT image showing medial osteochondral fracture (arrow).

Posterior impingement

- Posterior impingement develops secondary to repeated or forced ankle plantarflexion with subsequent compression of the soft tissues between the posterior process of the calcaneus and the tibia (Figs 7.14a, 7.15, 7.16).
- The lateral talar process or an os trigonum can also increase the degree of soft-tissue compression with or without stress reaction in the bone itself. The lateral process of the talus initially forms as a secondary ossification centre between the ages of 7 to 13 years and usually fuses with the main body of the talus. If there is a failure of fusion, the ossicle is known as an os trigonum and articulates with the talus via a synchondrosis (incidence 7 to 14%) (Fig. 7.14a). If the lateral talar process is unusually large or prominent it is sometimes termed a Steida process (Fig. 7.14b).
- The soft tissues compressed include the Kager's fat pad, tibiotalar capsule, posterior talofibular, intermalleolar and tibiofibular ligaments (Figs 7.15, 7.16). The flexor hallucis longus (FHL) tendon can also be secondarily involved although a primary tenosynovitis can clinically mimic posterior impingement.

Clinical features

- Posterior impingement is typically a chronic problem of insidious onset affecting athletes who regularly undergo forced plantarflexion, especially ballet dancers, jumping athletes, squash, and football players. Football players are particularly affected because plantarflexion occurs not only on push off during sprinting and changing direction but also during kicking.
- Symptoms include posterior ankle pain exacerbated by dorsiflexion or plantarflexion, which results in stretching or compression of the abnormal tissues.
- On examination there is posterior tibiotalar joint tenderness not involving the achilles tendon exacerbated by plantar flexion and dorsiflexion.
- Symptoms can also develop subacutely after an acute injury either posteriorly or elsewhere in the ankle and is not uncommon in football and ballet athletes who develop symptoms 4–6 weeks after a precipitating injury (Fig. 7.15).
- The precipitating acute injury leads to haemarthrosis and further synovial thickening which added to the background damage is enough to precipitate the syndrome.

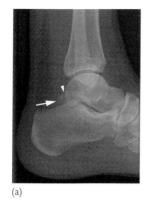

(a)

Fig. 7.14 (a) Os trigonum (arrow) and synchondrosis.

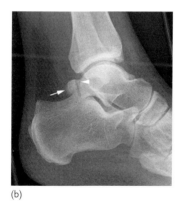

(b)

Fig. 7.14 (b) Steida process (arrow) and synchondrosis.

Imaging modalities

Radiography

Conventional radiographs can demonstrate an os trigonum or a Steida process, however these findings are commonly seen in asymptomatic individuals and minor stress fractures can be easily missed (Figs 7.14a, b).

Computed tomography (CT)

CT scanning can demonstrate more detailed bony anatomy including stress fractures, however soft tissue resolution is poor.

Magnetic resonance imaging (MRI)

- Conventional MR imaging is the optimal imaging modality as it can define bone marrow oedema, fracture lines or disruption of the synchondrosis indicating active bony impingement (Figs 7.15, 7.16).
- The ligaments are usually intact but surrounding posterior (particularly posterolateral) capsular oedema is commonly best seen on axial and sagittal T2-weighted sequences extending into Kager's fat pad (Fig. 7.16).
- Intravenous gadolinium can highlight small focal areas of enhancing synovitis around the posterior ligaments if oedema is not a predominating feature.
- MR imaging also allows accurate assessment of the remainder of the tibiotalar joint and surrounding tendons, which can aid treatment and surgical planning.
- If the abnormality is confirmed as focal with no other significant internal derangement on MR imaging, athletes can get good symptomatic relief after targeted ultrasound-guided injection of local anaesthetic and steroid into the nodular area (see below) (Fig. 7.16).

Management

- The majority of cases of posterior impingement of the ankle respond to conservative treatment (physiotherapy).
- Conventional MR imaging can define the degree of oedematous change and exclude concomitant abnormalities.
- Image-guided steroid and local anaesthetic injection into focal capsular thickening or the os trigonum synchondrosis provides long-lasting symptomatic relief in the majority of patients which can mean surgery is not required.
- A number of surgical studies have shown that arthroscopic resection of soft-tissue thickening and any associated bony abnormality with joint wash-out produces good symptomatic and functional results in resistant cases.

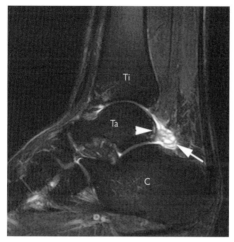

Fig. 7.15 Sagittal T2W MRI showing posterior synovitis (arrow) posterior talar (Ta) oedema (arrowhead). Note tibia (Ti) and calcaneus (c).

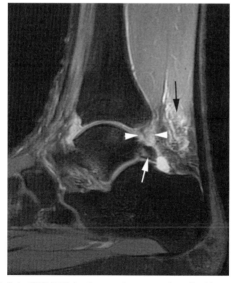

Fig. 7.16 Sagittal T2W MTI showing posterior synovitis (arrowheads), oedematous os trigonum (white arrow) and Kager's fat pad oedema.

Anterior impingement

Anterior ankle impingement is sometimes termed 'footballer's ankle'.

Pathogenesis

- The underlying mechanism of injury implicated is repeated supination injury which causes damage at the anteromedial margins of the articular cartilage.
- Other aetiological factors include repeated forced dorsiflexion (common in ballet and football) and direct microtrauma (particularly seen in football players during ball striking).
- Unlike other impingement syndromes osseous abnormality (anterior tibiotalar spurs) commonly forms a significant component of the impinging mass (Fig. 7.17a).
- Chronic damage to the chondral margins leads to repair with fibrous tissue, hyaline, and fibrocartilage undergoing subsequent enchondral ossification producing bone spurs.
- Studies of asymptomatic professional athletes have found a significant portion (>40%) to have anterior tibiotalar spurs on X-ray. It is thought that although these osseous abnormalities are an important part of this condition the development of additional capsular abnormality is critical for producing the clinical syndrome.

Clinical features

- Clinical features of this condition are anterior ankle pain with a subjective feeling of blocking on dorsiflexion.
- Examination reveals restrictive and painful dorsiflexion with occasionally palpable soft tissue swelling over the anterior joint.

Imaging modalities

Radiography

- Conventional radiographs are usually performed to confirm the extent and presence of osseous spurs on the lateral view (Fig. 7.17a).
- The tibiotalar spurs occur in typical positions at the anterior and medial articular cartilage margins.
- Radiographs also allow assessment of the remainder of the tibiotalar joint for secondary signs of degeneration including joint space reduction.

Magnetic resonance imaging (MRI)

- No significant radiology series evaluating cross-sectional imaging or ultrasound in this condition but MRI can deomonstrate the spurs and associated capsular thickening (Fig. 7.17b).

Management

- In athletes with anterior ankle impingement resistant to rehabilitative physiotherapy, arthroscopic resection of the osseous spurs and soft-tissue abnormality with joint wash-out has been shown to yield excellent functional and symptomatic results.

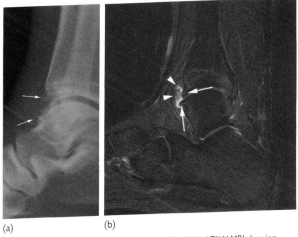

(a)
(b)

Fig. 7.17 (a) Anterior tibiotalar spurs (arrows). (b) Sagittal T2W MRI showing anterior tibiotalar spurs (arrows) and synovitis (arrowheads).

Anterolateral impingement

Pathogenesis

- Boundaries of the anterolateral ankle recess consist of the tibia posteromedially and fibula laterally with the tibiotalar joint capsule forming the anterior and lateral margins (Fig. 7.18).
- The capsule is reinforced by the anterior tibiofibular, anterior talofibular (Fig. 7.18) and calcaneofibular ligaments.
- Anterolateral impingement is thought to develop subsequent to a relatively minor injury usually consisting of forced ankle plantar flexion and supination.
- This injury mechanism generates tensile forces which tear the anterolateral capsular tissues without clinically significant mechanical instability. However, subsequent functional instability and associated repeated microtrauma can lead to further soft-tissue haemorrhage, synovial scarring and hypertrophy (Figs 7.19a, b).
- Ankle impingement syndromes can exist on their own or in combination with injuries such as chondromalacia and tendinopathy. It is important to recognize this clinically and radiologically so that coexistent pathologies are not missed resulting in potential treatment failure.

Clinical features

- Anterolateral ankle pain which is exacerbated on supination or pronation of the foot. Surgical series describe anterolateral tenderness, swelling, pain on single leg squat and pain on ankle dorsiflexion and eversion.

Imaging modalities

Magnetic resonance imaging (MRI)

- Conventional MR imaging has produced conflicting results in the pre-operative patient. Sensitivity and specificity for the detection of abnormality varies widely with an increase of accuracy occurring when a significant joint effusion is present (Fig. 7.19a).
- MR and CT arthrography studies have found a strong association between capsular irregularity of the anterolateral recess and subsequent surgical abnormality (Fig. 7.19b).
- The ligaments are usually not abnormal and soft tissue oedema is not commonly seen (unlike posterior impingement).

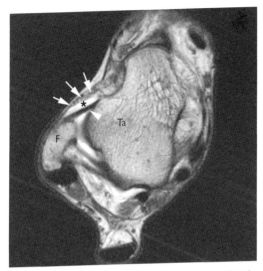

Fig. 7.18 Axial T2W MRI showing normal capsule (arrows), margin (*), and anterior talo fibular ligament (ATFL) (arrowhead). Note fibula (f) and talus (Ta).

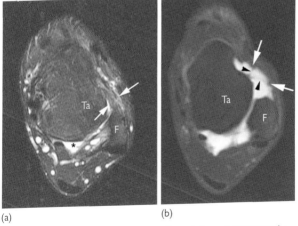

(a)   (b)

Fig. 7.19 (a) Axial T2W MRI showing thickened capsule (arrows). Note normal posterior capsule (*), fibula (f), and talus (Ta). (b) Axial T1W arthrogram showing thickened nodular capsule (arrows) and synechiae (arrowheads). Note fibula (f) and talus (Ta).

Ankle fractures

Ankle injuries are commonly seen in primary care and hospital accident departments.

- It is essential to determine extent of soft-tissue injury. This will determine stability of fracture. Generally, isolated non-displaced distal fibular or distal tibial fractures are stable in the absence of ligamentous instability.
- Medial injuries occur from eversion and abduction forces. The medial structures are the medial malleolus and the deltoid ligament. Avulsion of the distal medial malleolus occurs because the ligamentous strength is greater than the strength of the bone.
- Most unstable ankle fractures are the result of excessive external rotation of the talus with respect to the tibia. If the foot is supinated at the time of external rotation, an oblique fracture of the fibula ensues. If the foot is pronated at the time of external rotation, a mid- or high-fibular fracture results.
- Lateral injuries occur from inversion and adduction forces. The lateral structures are the distal fibula and the lateral ligaments of the ankle and subtalar joints.

Classification

The Weber classification is based on the level of the fracture in relationship to the joint mortice of the distal fibula.

- Type A fractures are horizontal avulsion fractures found below the mortice. They are stable and amenable to treatment with closed reduction and casting unless accompanied by a displaced medial malleolus fracture (Fig. 7.20).
- Type B fracture is a spiral fibular fracture that starts at the level of the mortice. These fractures may be stable or unstable depending on ligamentous injury or associated fractures on the medial side (Fig. 7.21a, b).
- Type C fracture is above the level of the mortise and disrupts the ligamentous attachment between the fibula and the tibia distal to the fracture. These fractures are unstable and require open reduction and internal fixation (Fig. 7.22).

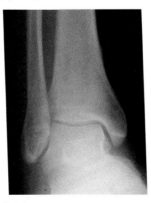

Fig. 7.20 Weber A fibula fracture.

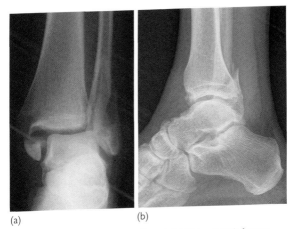

(a)   (b)

Fig. 7.21 (a) Weber B fibula fracture (AP view); (b) Weber B fibula fracture (lateral view).

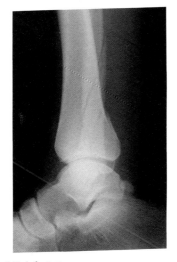

Fig. 7.22 Weber C fibula fracture.

Talar and calcaneal fractures

Talar fractures may occur as a result of severe trauma (e.g. motor vehicle accidents—the so-called 'aviator's talar fracture'), or through weight-bearing activities, typically sports.

- In severe trauma the neck of the talus is the most commonly involved site (Fig. 7.23 white arrow) although the body or head may be involved directly.
- Complete displacement may result in avascular necrosis of the talar body.
- Initial investigation is by plain film (AP and lateral views, supplemented with oblique, or Broden (45°) views). CT (coronal and axial views) is helpful to diagnose radiographically occult fractures (Fig. 7.24 white arrowhead).
- Avulsion injuries may occur around the margins of the talus, typically in the anterior region following forced dorsiflexion or at the posterior process with extreme plantarflexion.
- Osteochondral injuries may arise after acute sprains and dislocations even in the absence of fracture because of the relatively precarious blood supply to the talus. These are dealt more comprehensively with later in this chapter.

Calcaneal fractures usually occur due to trauma, typically the result of a fall or jump from height. Fatigue fractures are rare but may occur if in the presence of abnormal bone metabolism or if activity levels are exceptionally high.

- 25–30% of traumatic talar fractures are extra-articular.
- 70–75% are intra-articular, typically involving the subtalar joint.
- Several classification systems exist including Sander's, Rowe and Essex–Lopresti systems.
- Intra-articular fractures are often associated with secondary OA affecting the subtalar or calcaneocuboid joints. This should be considered in the patient who presents with persisting pain around the ankle and heel provoked by inversion/eversion of the heel.
- The primary fracture in compression injuries is more typically in the coronal plane at the level of the sinus tarsi. A range of secondary fracture lines can be seen and comminution into multiple fragments is not uncommon (Fig. 7.25).

Imaging modalities

Radiography
Plain film radiographs are usually acquired initially but may be unhelpful.

Computed tomography (CT)
CT investigations are definitive.

- Coronal views (angled perpendicular to the posterior facet) provide good visualization of the subtalar joint and the extension of fracture into the joint.
- Axial views provide good visualization of the calcaneocuboid and calcaneonavicular articulations.
- Scintigraphy (three-phase technetium[99] uptake scan) may be useful in differentiating fatigue fractures early.
- Primary traumatic fracture is most common with shear forces dividing the calcaneus into anteromedial and posterolateral fragments.

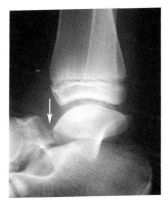

Fig. 7.23 Plain radiograph demonstrating displaced talar neck fracture.

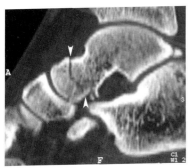

Fig.7.24 CT image of undisplaced talar neck fracture.

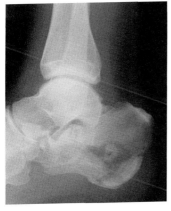

Fig. 7.25 Plain radiograph illustrating a comminuted calcaneal fracture.

Navicular and midfoot fractures

- Midfoot fractures may be traumatic or secondary to overuse.
- The navicular is a common site for stress fracture although diagnosis can be difficult as the fractures are often occult on plain radiographs.
- Less commonly the navicular can be involved in traumatic fractures. Traumatic fracture is usually associated with avulsion of the tuberosity although the body of the navicular may be involved if trauma is severe.

The most common presentation of a navicular fracture is as a stress reaction.

- Usually following a rapid increase in activity levels such as sporting participation (e.g. distance running) or long walks.
- Characterized by activity history, diffuse pain in the midfoot, exacerbation on activity and increasing intensity and localization of pain.
- The fracture is often preceded by intense bony oedema. Three-phase scintigraphy can help identify early stress reaction. MRI is useful for imaging stress fractures and is highly sensitive. Fig. 7.26 illustrates a severe stress fracture of the navicular with bone oedema and loss of cortical integrity in the upper third of the navicular articulation with the talus (white arrowhead).
- CT will typically show a breach of the cortex at the proximal, dorsal central one-third of the bone (Fig. 7.27 white arrowhead) which may propagate into the navicular body (Fig. 7.27 black arrows).

The most common traumatic fracture of the midfoot involves Lisfranc's joint (the tarsometatarsal joint). Subluxation of the Lisfranc joint may occur without fracture but all cases of Lisfranc joint derangement warrant a surgical consideration.

Usually any fracture is associated with dislocation of midfoot joints and, depending on the mechanism of injury, with a compression fracture of the calcaneus (nutcracker fracture). Common mechanisms of injury include stepping into a hole in the ground, trauma during sporting activities or traffic accidents.

The injury may be subtle to initial imaging especially if the injury is mainly ligamentous or if fractures are undisplaced. Subluxation is highly variable, ranging from isolated (e.g 1st metatarsal) displacement to full subluxation of the forefoot relative to the tarsal bones across the full width of the tarsometatarsal joint. Dorsal subluxation is more common than plantar subluxation. Severe injuries are obvious on plain film (Fig. 7.28 black arrows) but CT (Fig. 7.29) will be definitive.

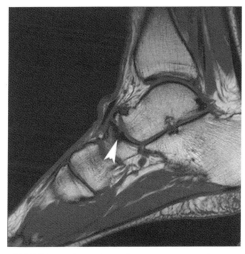

Fig. 7.26 T1W MRI coronal view showing hypointense region in the proximal navicular and a breach in the cortex.

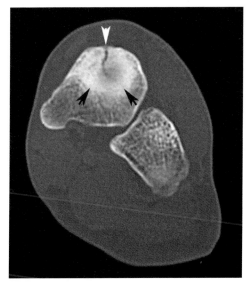

Fig. 7.27 Axial CT view showing typical stress fracture site and propagation in to the medulla.

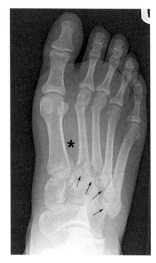

Fig. 7.28 AP plain film demonstrating multiple fracture sites at the bases of the lesser metatarsals.

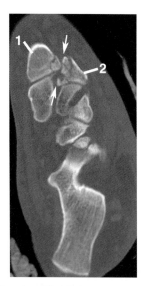

Fig. 7.29 Axial CT of complex midfoot fracture.

Metatarsal fractures

Traumatic fractures may affect any of the metatarsal bones.

- Usually readily diagnosed because of the long, slender structure of the metatarsals and the lack of confounding anatomy.
- AP, lateral and oblique films are adequate for traumatic fractures.
- The most common mechanism for traumatic fracture to a metatarsal is the dropping of a heavy object onto the forefoot.

A number of distinctive metatarsal fractures have also been described with relatively well-defined mechanisms of injury.

- Jones fracture—a transverse fracture occurring at the base of the 5th metatarsal immediately distal to the styloid process (Fig. 7.30 white arrows). The transverse Jones fracture should not be confused with the normal apophyseal line lying parallel to the long axis of the metatarsal in the skeletally immature foot. The most common presentation is secondarily to an inversion injury with or without ankle sprain although Jones fractures may occur in the absence of a clear history of trauma. Jones fractures remain undisplaced but care should be taken to identify full avulsion (pseudo-Jones) fractures.
- Less common is the dancer's fracture, also affecting the 5th metatarsal but presenting as a spiral fracture in the neck of the metatarsal. Dancer's fractures are usually associated with a highly specific mechanism of injury where a rotational force is applied to the foot while in full plantarflexion (such as dancing en pointe).
- 'March fractures' or metatarsal stress fractures are common and occur in response to repetitive excessive loading. They may occur as overuse fractures in response to high levels of sporting activity or as insufficiency fractures if bone density is reduced. The most common sites are the second, third and fifth metatarsals with the clinical presentation a diffuse pain in the affected region exacerbated by activity.

Imaging modalities

Radiography

- Frank fracture is usually not evident on plain film in the early stages
- Plain film may demonstrate callus formation and reparative activity in the healing stages (Fig. 7.31 white arrow).
- Scintigraphy has historically been the modality of choice but MRI (Fig. 7.32 white arrow) has high sensitivity and specificity to the changes seen in the early stress reaction and is now preferred where available.

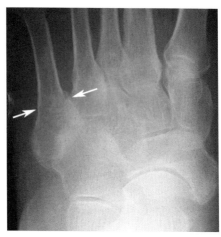

Fig. 7.30 AP plain film of a typical Jones fracture.

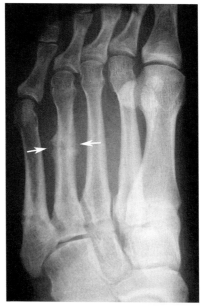

Fig. 7.31 Oblique radiograph of fracture and bony callus in the 4th metatarsal.

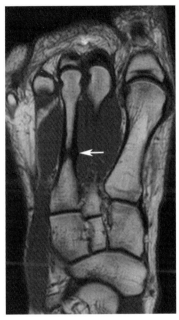

Fig. 7.32 T1W MRI demonstrating inflammation at the 4th metatarsal fracture site.

Intermetatarsal disorders

The three main intermetatarsal pathologies are intermetatarsal accessory bone, intermetatarsal bursitis, and Morton's neuroma.

Intermetatarsal accessory bones
- Relatively uncommon but can occur between the bases of the first and second metatarsals.
- Accessory bones at this site can be free-standing, articulating or fused.
- The presentation is of localized pain in the region.
- Accessory bones are visible on plain films although they require care to detect because of the complex local anatomy.

Intermetatarsal bursae
- Exist normally in each of the intermetatarsal spaces (Fig. 7.33 black arrows), lying superior to the deep transverse metatarsal ligament (arrow). They are anatomically discrete from the metatarsophalangeal joints.
- Intermetatarsal bursitis may occur secondary to systemic disease such as rheumatoid arthritis or because of local irritation.
- Inflammation within or distension of the bursae (bursitis) can cause forefoot pain. Severe bursitis can result in splaying of digits either side of the affected intermetatarsal space (the so-called 'daylight' sign).

Imaging modalities
Ultrasound (US)
Diagnostic ultrasound imaging is increasingly popular and offers a useful, alternative as displaceable structures such as bursae can be better visualized dynamically. Fig. 7.34 shows the extent (white arrows) a painful intermetatarsal bursa (white asterisk) extending out of the intermetatarsal space.

Magnetic resonance imaging (MRI)
Normal bursae can be difficult to identify on MR imaging except at high resolution but active bursitis is usually more obvious.

Morton's neuroma
- Not a true neuroma but a fibrotic enlargement of the perineureum, retaining a low signal intensity on T1- and T2-weighted MR sequences.
- Most often occurring in the 3rd/4th intermetatarsal space but can occur between any of the pairs of metatarsals.

Clinical features
- Clinical presentation is of pain, numbness or tingling in the affected interdigital cleft and the associated toes. Pain may radiate proximally or onto the plantar aspect of the forefoot. Symptoms are exacerbated by standing or walking, especially in narrow or high-heeled shoes. Relief is obtained by rest and by massage of the affected region.
- 'Mulder's click' elicited by lateral compression has long been considered diagnostic although the click can be reproduced in normal feet.

Imaging modalities
Ultrasound (US)
Differentiation of Morton's neuroma and intermetatarsal bursitis can be made readily with MRI but more recently, diagnostic ultrasound has

offered a viable alternative. The diagnosis of Morton's using ultrasound is operator-dependent and care must be taken to expose the deep-lying neuroma (Fig. 7.35a) adequately through lateral or dorsal compression (Fig. 7.35b asterix).

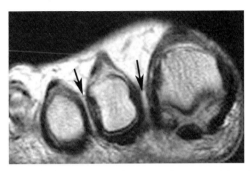

Fig. 7.33 T1W MIR demonstrating normal anatomy at the metatarsophalangeal joints.

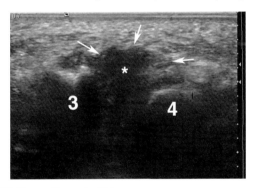

Fig. 7.34 Ultrasound image of an IM bursa.

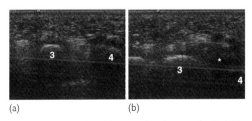

(a) (b)

Fig. 7.35 Ultrasound images of an IM neuroma lying between the third (3) and fourth (4) metatarsal (a) before and (b) after lateral compression.

Gout

Two main types:
- acute gout (podagra)
- chronic (often tophaceous) gout

Acute gout

Points to consider:
- Main differential is infection—aspiration allows this to be ruled out and crystal synovitis to be confirmed.
- Typical site for gout is first metatarsophalangeal joint but any joint in the foot and ankle can be involved.
- Systemic symptoms such as fever may occur.
- Inflammatory markers, such as C reactive protein (CRP), may be markedly elevated. Serum uric acid may be normal in acute attack.
- Some treatments cause an increase in the serum uric acid and may predispose to gout. These include thiazide diuretics and low dose aspirin. Alcohol (particularly beer) and high purine diet also risk factors.
- Raised uric acid is a risk factor for cardiovascular disease and often associated with obesity, alcohol, high lipids, hypertension (metabolic syndrome)

Chronic (tophaceous) gout

- May occur insidiously
- Is often polyarticular—large and small joints
- Same risk factors as in acute gout
- Much more likely to be associated with abnormalities on plain X-ray. Erosions are juxta-articular and punched out ('rat-bite erosions')
- Tophi may occur in Achilles tendon

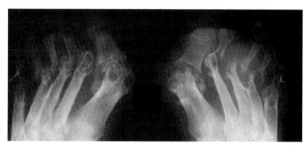

Fig. 7.36 Plain radiograph of feet demonstrating 'punched-out' or 'rat-bite' erosions (arrows) typical of gout.

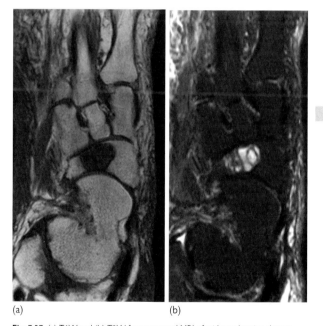

(a)   (b)

Fig. 7.37 (a) T1W and (b) T2W fat suppressed MRI of mid-tarsal region demonstrating intra-osseous tophi (arrows).

Inflammatory arthritis of the forefoot

Inflammatory arthritis of the forefoot frequently presents with pain under the metatarsal heads and the complaint of 'walking on pebbles'. Persistent synovitis of the metatarsophalangeal joints leads to both articular and soft-tissue damage, possibly because it is difficult to advise people with inflammation in these joints that they should not expose them to significant loading. Common diseases causing inflammation of the forefoot:
- Rheumatoid arthritis
- Psoriatic arthritis, reactive arthritis and other spondyloarthropathies
- Miscellaneous conditions such as sarcoidosis

Rheumatoid arthritis
- 90% of people with rheumatoid arthritis have forefoot involvements
- Persistent synovitis in metatarsophalangeal joints causes erosion and destruction of the joints (Fig. 7.38)
- Associated involvement of the ligamentous tissues which maintain the integrity of the forefoot leads to splaying of the forefoot, migration of the metatarsal fat pad and ventral subluxation of the metatarsal heads
- Callus forms under the metatarsal heads and an adventitious bursa forms between the callus and metatarsal head. The bursa may became inflamed and subsequently ulcerate through the callus
- Interphalangeal joint involvement leads to deformity, usually hammer and claw toes, the dorsal surface of which may ulcerate due to friction with footwear
- Synovitis of the metatarsophalangeal joints may simulate Morton's neuroma (see Fig. 7.39)
- Nodules and vasculitis may occur on the toes and represent extra-articular involvement

Psoriatic arthritis, reactive arthritis and the spondyloarthropathies
- Inflammation of metatarsophalangeal and interphalangeal joints is more patchy and less symmetrical (Fig. 7.40).
- Inflammation of interphalangeal joint of the great toe may occur in isolation.

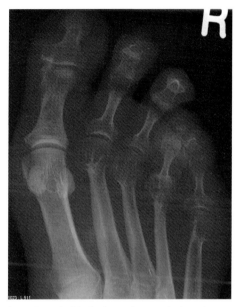

Fig. 7.38 Plain radiograph of the forefoot in rheumatoid arthritis demonstrating erosions of the metatarsal heads.

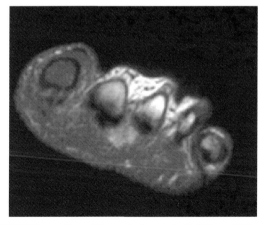

Fig. 7.39 MR image with gadolinium contrast demonstrating high signal in the second and third metatarso-phalangeal joints with inter-metatarsal bursitis.

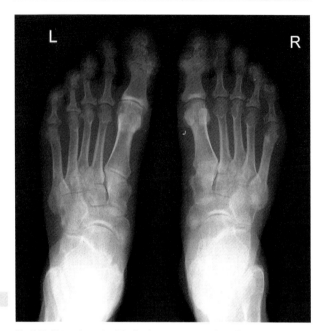

Fig. 7.40 Plain radiograph of the forefoot in psoriatic arthritis demonstrating patchy arthritis of the small joints of the foot. The inter-phalangeal joint of the right great toe demonstrates marked peri-articular new bone formaxon, typical of this disorder.

It may be possible to distinguish isolated distal interphalangeal joint inflammation.

- Dactylitis (sausage digit) occurs most commonly in the 4th toe. Dactylitis involves inflammation of all the tissues of the digit with both articular, osseous and soft-tissue inflammation (Fig. 7.41)
- Nail involvement (onycholysis, hyperkeratosis, and pitting) may be present as well as psoriaform lesions on the foot

Miscellaneous conditions such as sarcoidosis

- Musculoskeletal sarcoidosis can present with pain and swelling of a toe, resembling dactylitis
- Lupus pernio and pulmonary involvement provide support for this diagnosis
- Plain radiography shows a lacy pattern of bone in the phalangeal shaft (Fig. 7.42)

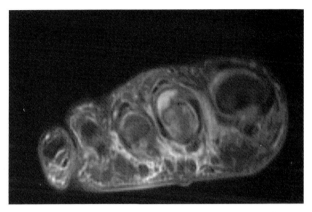

Fig. 7.41 MR with gadolinium contrast in psoriatic arthritis with dactylitis of the second toe. Note bone oedema and both flexor and extensor tenosynovitis.

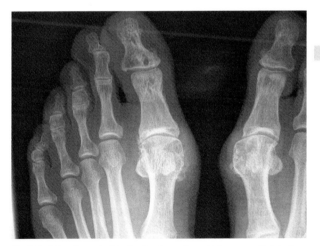

Fig. 7.42 Plain radiograph of the forefoot in a patient with bone sarcoidosis in the left great toe. Note the 'lacy' pattern of the bone trabeculae in the distal phalanx.

Hallux rigidus and hallux valgus

- Hallux rigidus and hallux valgus are named classifications from a spectrum of pathologies affecting the first metatarsophalangeal joint.
- Both hallux rigidus and hallux valgus are acquired deformities resulting from a complex combination of inherited factors and extrinsic and intrinsic mechanical factors.

Hallux rigidus

- The first metatarsophalangeal joint becomes progressively fixed but without significant deformity in the coronal or transverse planes.
- In the early stages the joint may demonstrate progressive limitation of movement and is therefore sometimes described as hallux limitus.
- Radiologically, the findings are typical of osteoarthritic change. Prior to full fusion (i.e. onset of true hallux rigidus) movement of the joint may be painful because of physical limitation of dorsiflexion range due to osteophyte formation (Fig. 7.43 white arrow) and inflammation as evidenced by the power Doppler signal in Fig. 7.43 (white arrowheads).
- In the later stages, degenerative changes predominate, with loss of joint space, periarticular osteophyte formation and subchondral sclerosis evident at affected joints (Fig. 7.44 white arrows).

Hallux valgus

- Describes a deformity of the first metatarsophalangeal joint wherein the hallux is deviated toward the midline of the foot with or without axial (valgus) rotation.
- The first metatarsophalangeal joint undergoes similar histological changes to those seen hallux limitus/rigidus but with angular deformity overlaid.

The diagnosis is normally made clinically although radiographic investigation is helpful in preoperative planning and may be used to quantify baseline and postoperative deformity.

Imaging modalities

Radiography

- Plain film radiography, using AP, lateral and oblique views is adequate to visualize the relationship between the hallux and the metatarsal (Fig. 7.45).
- Non-weight-bearing radiographs have long been the standard although standing (weigh-tbearing) views are now considered preferable.
- The normal angle formed between the long axis of the hallux and the metatarsal is 10–14° dependent on the specific technique used. A diagnosis of hallux valgus may be considered if this angle exceeds 20–25° although grading systems usually incorporate clinical findings.
- Other radiographic signs can include a prominent dorsomedial osteophyte with an associated bursa (the bunion), subluxation of the sesamoid bones toward the midline of the foot, subluxation of the proximal phalanx on the metatarsal head and secondary adduction of the metatarsal on the medial cuneiform.

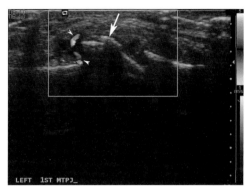

Fig. 7.43 Ultrasound image with power Doppler shopwing a dorsal osteophyte and local inflammation at a pathological first metatarsophalangeal joint.

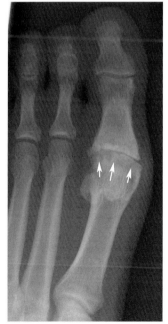

Fig. 7.44 Plain radiograph of hallux rigidus showing loss of joint space.

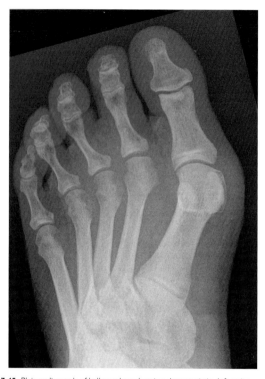

Fig. 7.45 Plain radiograph of hallux valgus showing characteristic deformity.

Diabetic foot (Charcot's arthropathy and osteomyelitis)

The presentation of joint disease in the patient with diabetes may be complicated by a number of factors including impaired sensation, associated ulceration, predisposition to infection, and autonomic impairment.

- Concomitant osteoarthritis of foot joints is to be expected in many older people regardless of diabetes status and so arthropathy may also be independent of systemic disease.
- Neuropathy in long-standing, poorly controlled diabetes can contribute to a characteristic joint degeneration, Charcot's arthropathy, where damage is severe and wide ranging. In advanced disease the diagnosis is straightforward but in early disease signs may be subtle.
- The presence of foot ulceration and raised blood glucose may predispose the diabetic patient to osteomyelitis and infective arthritis and these differentials must be considered when imaging the diabetic foot.

Charcot's arthropathy

- Initial presentation is usually of a slightly swollen, warm joint, typically in the midfoot and associated with loss of function and/or progressing, but at this stage mild, deformity.
- Pain is absent or reduced relative to what might be expected, because of the associated neuropathy.
- As large fracture fragments are re-absorbed the arthropathy enters a coalescent phase. Finally ankylosis of remaining fragments and hypertrophy of new bone formation result a reconstructive phase where a pseudo-joint is created, often with considerable residual deformity.

Imaging modalities

Radiography

- Plain films are not especially helpful early as initial changes mimic those of the more benign osteoarthritis.

Magnetic resonance imaging (MRI)

- MR investigation or three-phase scintigraphy can identify areas of active bone disease prior to structural change, with bone marrow oedema occurring in the earliest stages. Note that these techniques are not specific and cannot differentiate readily between neuropathic, osteomyelitic, neoplastic and inflammatory processes.
- New approaches such as Indium[111] labelled leukocyte scintigraphy offer better differentiation between infected and neuropathic joints, but such techniques are not yet used routinely.
- As the Charcot's arthropathy becomes more established, the marrow signal on MRI becomes heterogeneous. Around the affected region there is wide-ranging osseous destruction and dislocation (Fig. 7.46a, b). These are also clearly visible on plain radiographs.

Osteomyelitis is readily treatable in its early stages and every effort should be made to exclude the presence of infection. Bearing in mind the difficulties in differentiating osteomyelitic change from a developing Charcot's joint, ruling out treatable osteomyelitic infection should be considered a priority over establishing a firm diagnosis of Charcot's arthropathy.

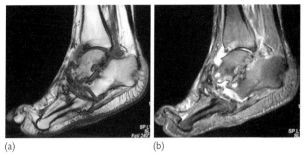

(a)   (b)

Fig 7.46 (a) and (b) T2W of an advanced Charcot joint illustrating widespread joint destruction.

Pseudotumours

- Foreign body granulomas are not uncommon and a correlating traumatic history can be frequently absent.
- Imaging usually consists of radiographs but these can miss non-opaque foreign bodies. In this situation ultrasound is still effective in detecting an echogenic body amongst hypoechoic granulomatous tissue (Fig. 7.47).
- Morton's neuroma is discussed elsewhere in this chapter.

Soft tissue and osseous tumours

- The ankle and foot is a relatively rare area for any specific osseous or soft-tissue tumours.
- True neuromas and vascular malformations not infrequently occur in this region but are more commonly seen elsewhere (Fig. 7.48).
- Plantar fibromas (Ledderhose's disease) are a common clinical condition and are benign fibromatous tumours of the deep plantar fascia, extending into the subcutaneous fat and less commonly the deeper tissues (Figs 7.49a, b).
- They are histologically identical to fibromas found in the palmar aponeurosis of the hand.
- They can be frequently multiple and bilateral (20–50%). They are concomitant with palmar lesions in 50%. They also have an increased incidence in patients with diabetes, epilepsy, and alcohol-induced cirrhosis of the liver.
- They can be painful but frequently are asymptomatic with patients concerned about appearances or difficulty in fitting footwear.

Imaging modalities

Imaging evaluation can be by MR imaging or ultrasound (Figs 7.49a, b). The fibroma can appear heterogeneous on ultrasound, Doppler ultrasound and T2-weighted MR imaging. However, its origin from the fascia and well-defined margins with the subcutaneous fat are characteristic and reassuring.

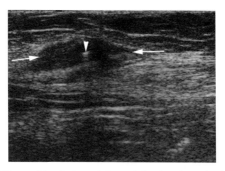

Fig. 7.47 Ultrasound showing hypoechoic granulation tissue (arrows) and echogenic foreign body (arrowhead).

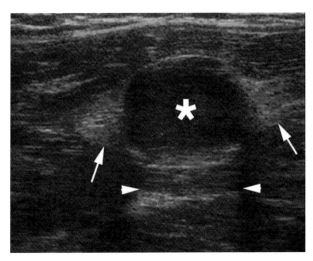

Fig. 7.48 Ultrasound showing hypoechoic neuroma (*), with tail sign (arrows) and distal acoustic enhancement (arrowheads).

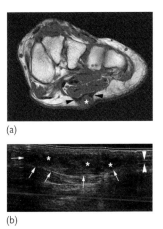

(a)

(b)

Fig. 7.49 (a) Coronal T1W MRI showing plantar fascia (arrowheads) and fibroma (*). (b) Ultrasound showing normal adjacent plantar fascia (arrowheads), fibroma (arrows) and hypoechoic vacuoles within (*).

Achilles tendon

The Achilles tendon can undergo traumatic or degenerative damage. The normal tendo Achilles is oval in cross section and fairly consistent in diameter from the myotendinous junction to its insertion (Fig. 7.50a). The Achilles tendon is not invested in a synovial sheath and so tenosynovitis is never seen.

Achilles tendonosis

- Presents as a thickening of the tendon body usually in a zone 4–8cm proximal to the insertion where the blood supply is poor.
- The usually compact arrangement of tendon fibres is lost and the tendon can become heterogeneous on ultrasound or MR imaging.
- A fusiform swelling may be evident both clinically and on imaging (Fig. 7.50b). Within this region small longitudinal, or less commonly, transverse tears can sometimes be seen.

Imaging modalities

- MR is highly sensitive to partial tears (Fig. 7.51 white arrow), ultrasound less so, although power Doppler signal may be demonstrated. Localized calcinosis may be present in long-standing pathology.

Tears

- Partial tears of insidious onset are common in degenerate tendons and may progress to full-thickness tears (Fig. 7.52). Acute trauma, however, can result in partial or full thickness tears of the tendo Achilles even in normal tendons.
- Traumatic tears usually occur during rapid, unexpected dorsiflexion such as tripping on a step, or during unaccustomed activity such as a sudden return to sports.

Other retrocalcaneal symptoms

- Achilles tendonosis should not be confused with retrocalcaneal bursitis.
- Inflammation of the bursa interposed between the tendon and upper calcaneus can present with a similar clinical picture.
- Clinical differentiation can be made by direct pressure to determine whether any effusion can be displaced.

Imaging modalities

Magnetic resonance imaging (MRI)

- MR or ultrasound imaging is usually readily diagnostic. An actively inflamed bursa will yield a hyperintense signal on T2-weighted MR sequences or power Doppler signal at ultrasound examination.

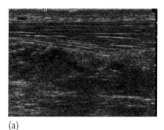

(a)

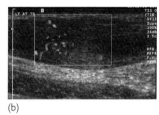

(b)

Fig. 7.50 Ultrasound of Achilles tendon showing (a) normal structure and (b) the characteristic fusiform swelling indicating tendonopathy (with power Doppler evidence of increased vascularity).

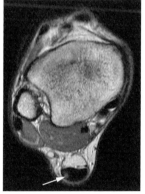

Fig. 7.51 T2W MRI showing a hyperintense signal at the site of a partial tear.

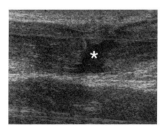

Fig. 7.52 Ultrasound shows complete tear of the Achilles tendon with free fluid (*) between the ends.

Plantar fascia

- Several underlying processes are implicated in the syndrome commonly ascribed to pathology of the plantar fascia.
- Clinically it can be difficult to differentiate between causes of pain in the plantar heel area and so imaging is often useful.

Common causes of plantar heel pain include:
- Fat pad atrophy
- Contusion
- Heel spur
- Nerve entrapment
- Epiphysitis (in adolescence)
- Stress fracture

The presence of a heel spur on plain films or other imaging is an unreliable finding, with many being asymptomatic.

Clinical features

The presentation of pain in the region of the plantar fascia is usually termed 'plantar fasciitis' clinically, although inflammation is rarely seen and the term fasciosis is probably more applicable.
- The history is of plantar heel pain immediately distal to the medial calcaneal tubercle, usually worse on first weight-bearing.
- The pain can radiate into the medial longitudinal arch and is sometimes precipitated during the examination by dorsiflexion of the foot and the toes.

Imaging modalities

Magnetic resonance imaging (MRI)

- Sagittal T1-weighted MRI sequences will show a thickened plantar fascia but inflammation is minimal on T2-weighted images. Enhancement may show local oedema but does not aid diagnosis.

Ultrasound (US)

- The same thickening is also evident on ultrasonography (typically to greater than 4mm (Figs. 7.53a, b white arrowheads) and this method is preferred by many.
- In unilateral cases comparison with the asymptomatic side is helpful and will aid in both gauging the extent of thickening and in determining whether the affected plantar fascia is hypoechogenic, another indicator of pathology.
- Other findings at sonography might include peri-fascial oedema and intra-substance calcinosis.

Frank rupture may occur, typically following repeat steroid injection, but is rare.

Nodular thickening of the plantar fascia such as seen in Ledderhose's disease (plantar fibromatosis) 📖 Soft tissue and osseous tumours, p.248.

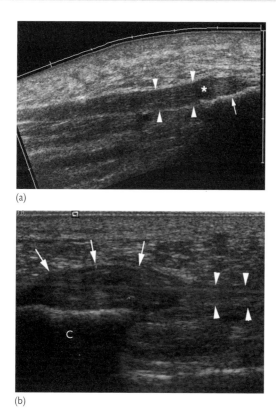

(a)

(b)

Fig. 7.53 (a) Ultrasound of plantar fascia thickening (arrowheads), focal loss of echotexture (*) near origin (arrow) with partial longitudinal tear; (b) marked thickening (arrows) at calcaneus (c) with more normal structure distally (arrowheads).

Chapter 8

Investigating spinal problems

Anatomy

Embryology

The vertebral column and the associated musculature develop from the paraxial mesenchyme which is found lateral to the notochord and neural tube in early embryonal development. The paraxial mesenchyme undergoes segmentation and then somitogenesis sequentially in a craniocaudal direction. The sclerotomal cells from each somite enclose the notochord and together form the blastemal centrum of each vertebra. Neural processes extend from the dorsal aspect of the centrum to encase the neural tube. The neural arch consists of the paired bilateral pedicles, laminae and spinous processes. The definitive vertebral body is formed by the blastemal centrum anteriorly and the expanding pedicles posterolaterally which fuse at the neurocentral synchondrosis. The notochord lying between the vertebral bodies forms the nucleus pulposus while the mesenchyme surrounding it forms the annulus fibrosis.

The occipito–cervical junction however develops from the occipital sclerotomes. The development of the upper cervical spine is therefore more closely related to the basiocciput, and anomalous developments therefore often affect both these regions together.

Ossification

Each vertebra typically ossifies from three primary ossification centres: one for the centrum and one each for each half of the neural arch. Ossification centres appear as early as 9 weeks of gestation. The arches unite posteriorly typically between 1 and 3 years of age while the centrum unites with the arches at the neurocentral synchondrosis between 3 and 6 years of age. This process progresses cranio-caudally.

The upper two cervical vertebrae have a different pattern of ossification to the typical vertebra described above.

At puberty, five secondary ossification centres (Fig. 8.1) appear: one for each transverse process; one for the spinous process; and two ring apophyses for the circumferential parts of the upper and lower surfaces of the vertebral bodies which form the vertebral endplates. These secondary centres usually fuse by 17–18 years of age.

There are significant biomechanical forces acting at the apophyses where there are muscular and ligamentous attachments. These sites are therefore prone to injuries in children, prior to fusion.

Bones

The spinal column is composed of 31 to 33 vertebrae: 7 cervical, 12 thoracic, 5 lumbar, 5 sacral and 3–4 coccygeal segments. The individual sacral and coccygeal vertebrae are usually fused together with almost no motion between the individual segments.

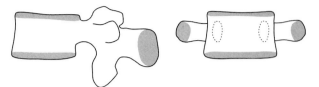

Fig. 8.1 Secondary ossification centres. Figure shows the five secondary centres of ossification (shaded areas) in a typical vertebra (one each at the superior and inferior aspect of the vertebral body also called the ring apophyses, one each for each transverse process and one for the spinous process).

Joints of the spine (Fig. 8.2)

The joints include the intervertebral disc (IVD), facet joints and in the cervical spine, uncovertebral joints.

The IVD is the major joint through out the spinal column. The disc is composed of central gelatinous nucleus pulposus and the peripheral annulus fibrosis which is arranged in a fashion similar to a concentric 'onion skin' arrangement around the nucleus.

Each vertebra typically has two facets posteriorly on each side of the midline each of which have superior and inferior articular facets. The superior facet of each vertebra articulates with the inferior facet of the vertebra above to form the synovial facet joints. The alignment of the facet joints varies in different parts of the spinal column (coronally in the cervical spine and thoracic spine becoming sagitally orientated in the lumbar spine) to allow movements in certain directions while restricting movements in other directions (principally rotation in the cervical and thoracic spine and flexion extension in the lumbar spine).

The uncovertebral joints are specific to the cervical spine and are formed on the lateral aspect of the disc by the uncinate process of one vertebra with the concavity seen in the adjacent vertebra. These synovial joints are not present at birth and form in childhood. These joints are susceptible to degeneration with age and are a principal cause of morbidity along with disc degeneration as osteophytes from these joints narrow the exit foramina of the cervical nerves.

Ligaments

There are a number of ligaments in the spinal column. The anterior longitudinal ligament runs along the anterior borders of the vertebrae from the craniocervical junction to the lumbosacral junction and is closely applied to the vertebral bodies and the disc. The posterior longitudinal ligament (PLL) runs along the posterior margins of the vertebrae and runs from the level of C2 to the sacrum and is only loosely adherent to the vertebrae and the disc. Beyond the C2 cranially, the PLL continues as the tectorial membrane and attaches to the anterolateral aspects of the foramen magnum. The ligamentum flavum extends from the lamina of one vertebra to the lamina of the adjacent vertebra on either side of the midline and forms the dorsal aspect of the spinal canal. The interspinous ligament extends from the spinous process of one vertebra to the spinous process of the adjacent vertebra. The supraspinous ligament connects the tips of the spinous processes.

There is a complex array of ligaments at the craniocervical junction (Fig. 8.3) to allow the complex rotational movements at this site. These include the anterior and posterior atlanto–occipital membranes, the cruciate ligament with its vertical and horizontal (transverse) components, apical ligament and the alar ligaments. The alar ligaments are important and restrict the head rotation to the opposite side. Similarly the transverse ligament helps to control anterior translation of the atlas with respect to the axis.

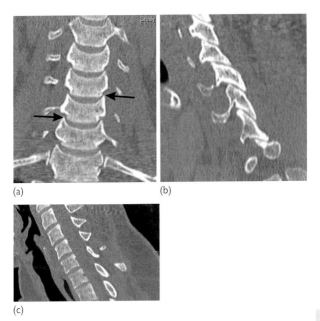

Fig. 8.2 Joints: reformatted CT images show (a) uncovertebral joints (unique to the cervical region, marked by black arrows), (b) facet joints, and (c) discovertebral joint.

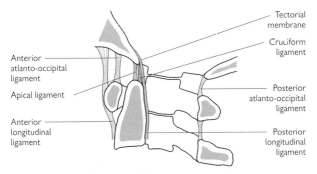

Fig. 8.3 Ligaments at the craniocervical junction.

Disc degeneration

Pathogenesis

The disc, in particular the nucleus pulposus, is rich in proteoglycans and has a collagen matrix. The proteoglycans provide a high osmotic content and pressure in the nucleus pulposus. In young people, the nucleus consists of approximately 90% water and the annulus contains 80% water.

Ageing results in dehydration and loss of resilience in the disc and involves the neighbouring bone (intervertebral osteochondrosis—see Fig. 8.4). The nucleus becomes dessicated and friable with loss of the normal onion-skin appearance of the nucleus, clefts appear, there is loss of disc height and bone marrow changes in the adjacent endplate result in oedema, fatty infiltration, and finally sclerosis. There is nitrogen collection in the disc space, the so-called 'vacuum phenomenon'. This is exacerbated in extension (due to negative pressure in the disc) and reduced in flexion.

Disc dehydration occurs in all adults to a certain degree even as early as the second decade of life. This process is physiological and only considered pathological when accelerated.

The endplate and adjacent marrow respond to the degeneration and are seen as Modic changes.

The hallmark of spondylosis deformans (Fig. 8.5) is osteophyte formation, particularly along the lateral and anterior aspect of the spine. The initial insult is thought to be disruption of the outer (Sharpey's) fibres of the annulus, the disc protrudes anteriorly and lifts the attachment of the anterior longitudinal ligament producing osteophytes as a response to mechanical stress.

Patients present with pain, stiffness, and limitation of movement.

Imaging modalities

Radiology

Findings include vacuum phenomenon, loss of disc height, endplate sclerosis, Schmorl's nodes (intraosseous disc herniation). Most common in the lower lumbar and cervical regions. Radiographs insensitive until morphological changes occur.

The osteophytes of spondylosis deformans occur several millimetres away from the corner of the vertebra, initially extend horizontally before turning vertically and may eventually bridge the disc space. This helps distinguish them from syndesmophytes 📖 see p. 298.

Magnetic resonance imaging (MRI)

Earlier identification of degeneration compared to other imaging modalities. However, changes in signal intensity of disc occur with advancing age universally and are difficult to differentiate from pathological degeneration. The earliest feature is a decrease in signal intensity in the nucleus pulposus corresponding to loss of hydration. Vacuum phenomenon is seen as linear areas of signal void on both T1W and T2W images. Calcification in the disc also seen as signal void.

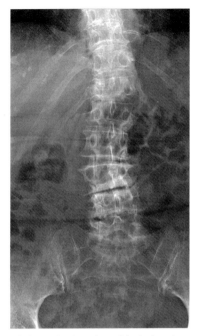

Fig. 8.4 Intervertebral osteochondrosis. Loss of disc height and vacuum phenomenon.

Changes in the endplates are manifested as Modic changes:
- type 1 (fibrovascular reaction)—low signal on T1W and high signal on T2W, enhancement with gadolinium
- type II (fatty marrow)—high signal on both T1W and T2W images;
- type III (bone sclerosis)—low signal on both T1W and T2W images.

Annular tears are commonly seen on MRI (significance unclear but occur more frequently in people with back pain).

Imaging modalities

Computed tomography (CT)

Disc height loss, endplate sclerosis, osteophytes. Useful to differentiate vacuum phenomenon from calcification seen on MRI.

Differential diagnosis

Infection (rapidly progressive loss of disc height, sclerosis, poorly defined vertebral end plate outlines, and sometimes a soft tissue mass). The vacuum phenomenon (highly specific for degenerative disease) is a particularly useful sign. *Neoplasms* do not usually involve disc space directly. *Diffuse idiopathis skeletal hyperostosis* (DISH)—extensive ossification along the lateral and anterior aspects of the vertebral column. Associated ligamentous calcification and ossification elsewhere.

Ankylosing spondylitis (AS) produces ossification of the outer annular fibres resulting in syndesmophytes which are typically thin and vertically oriented. Involvement of the sacroiliac, apophyseal and costoverterbal articulations is seen in AS.

Psoriasis and Reiter's disease can produce syndesmophytes, initially separate from the spinal surface, poorly defined and of irregular contour. Osteophytes can also be produced in hypoparathyroidism, paralysis, vitamin A excess and fluorosis.

Complications

Osteophytes can cause dysphagia, pain, restricted motion. Nucleus pulposus displacement resulting in disc prolapsed and radicular pain.

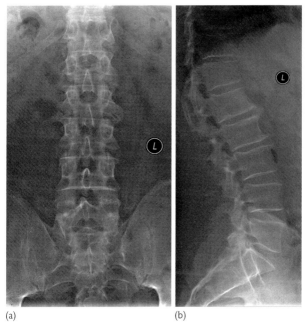

(a)   (b)

Fig. 8.5 Spondylosis deformans. Osteophytes are noted at the L2/3 level and are oriented horizontally.

Complications of disc degeneration

Disc prolapse (Fig. 8.6)

The disc can displace in any direction: superiorly or inferiorly (causing Schmorl's nodes), anteriorly (causing spondylosis deformans) or posteriorly (intraspinal herniation).

The terminology to indicate the various patterns of posterior disc displacement/herniation:

- *Bulge*—intact annular fibres with a diffuse pattern of disc displacement of >180° circumference, beyond the contours of the vertebral body
- *Protrusion*—the nucleus displaces focally (<180°) through some of the annular fibres but is still confined by the intact outermost annular fibres
- *Extrusion*—the nucleus penetrates all the annular fibres and lies underneath the posterior longitudinal ligament
- *Sequestration*—there is discontinuity between the displaced nucleus and the parent disc. The disc fragment may herniate through the PLL and lie in the epidural space or displace underneath the PLL to a variable distance from the parent disc.

Clinical features

Radiculopathy (pain, paraesthesia in the distribution of a nerve root with associated motor or sensory deficit), spinal stenosis (claudication after a few yards relieved by rest and flexion).

Imaging modalities

Magnetic resonance imaging (MRI)

Best imaging modality to depict direction, degree and severity of disc displacement and its effects on neurological structures. Sequestrated fragment can migrate in any direction and can be seen a significant distance away from the originating disc. They usually demonstrate higher T2W signal compared to the nucleus pulposus of the parent disc, which may be related to the hydrophilic properties of the disc. Sequestered disc fragments can also completely regress with time.

Computed tomography (CT)

CT demonstrates the disc prolapse but does not identify individual neurological structures directly. This can be achieved by intrathecal iodinated contrast administration (CT myelography). CT and MRI show degree of stenosis and effects on neurological structures.

Differential diagnosis

Intravenous gadolinium administration useful to differentiate epidural tumours from disc and also to differentiate scarring from recurrent disc after previous discectomy.

Segmental instability

Spinal mobility is complex and is dependant on a number of factors including integrity of disc, apophyseal joints, orientation of the facet joints, spinal curvature, ligaments and muscles.

Radiographs

Flexion, neutral and extension radiographs reveal spondylolisthesis or retrolisthesis, change in the disc height, abrupt change in the length of the pedicles, narrowing of intervertebral foramina, malalignment of spinous processes, abrupt change in interspinous distance, abrupt change in angulation between adjacent spinal segments.

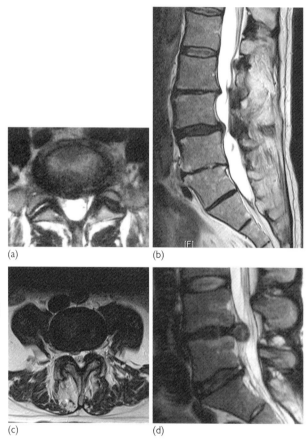

(a)   (b)

(c)   (d)

Fig. 8.6 Various forms of disc prolapse. Axial T2W MRI (a) shows a generalized expansion of the disc in keeping with a disc bulge with intact annulus. Sagittal (b) and axial (c) T2W images show a small focal protrusion of the nucleus pulposus with intact annulus fibrosis. Sagittal (d) and axial *(cont.)*

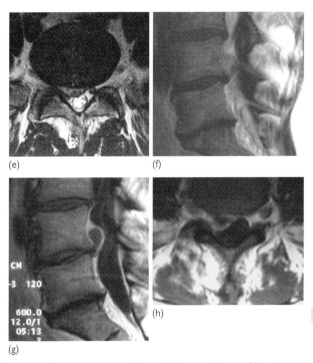

Fig. 8.6 (Cont.) (e) T2W MRI shows nucleus extrusion through the full thickness of the annulus and lying underneath the posterior longitudinal ligament. Sagittal T2W MRI (f) shows high signal intensity mass adjacent but separate to the L4/5 disc extending behind the L4 vertebra. This mass does not demonstrate any enhancement on the sagittal (g) and axial (h) post-contrast MRIs in keeping with a disc sequestration.

Spondylolisthesis and degenerative listhesis

Forward displacement of one vertebra over a contiguous vertebra is termed spondylolisthesis. This may be degenerative, spondylolytic (isthmic) or more rarely due to other causes.

Degenerative spondylolisthesis is caused by degenerative disease of the facet joints with associated disc degeneration. This may be primary or secondary to inflammatory arthritis.

Prevalence

Commonest cause of spondylolisthesis >50 years of age (5%) and usually affects the lower lumbar spine (L4/5 commonly). Can also involve the cervical spinal canal. More common in women (4:1) and people of African origin (3:1).

Pathology

The degeneration and hypertrophy in the facet joints along with the laxity in the capsule allows excess motion at the facet joints which in turn results in translation of one vertebral body with respect to the other. This also results in buckling of the overlying ligamentum flavum. The combination of features results in narrowing of spinal canal. When severe, this can cause thecal sac and neurological compression.

The AP diameter of the superior surface of the lower vertebra is divided into four quarters to grade spondylolisthesis (grades I–IV are assigned to slips of one, two, three or four quarters of the lower vertebral diameter respectively as seen on the lateral radiograph).

Clinical features

Pain worse on extension and relieved by stooping forward. Unilateral or bilateral facet joint pain at the level of degeneration. Spinal claudication (bilateral leg pain, numbness, weakness worse during walking/standing/extension, relieved in the supine position/flexion) secondary to spinal canal stenosis. Radicular pain due to nerve root compression. Cord or cauda equina compression may ensue.

Imaging modalities

Radiographs (Fig. 8.7)

Demonstrate the anterior translation of one vertebra over the adjacent inferior vertebra. Flexion extension radiographs may demonstrate instability. Facet joint degeneration is seen as sclerosis and hypertrophy of the facet joints. Spinal canal narrowing can be seen as reduced anteroposterior dimension of the affected level compared to the adjacent levels (<13mm in cervical spine and <16mm in lumbar spine). Measurements are not, however, accurate indicators of disease severity. The spinolaminar junction is also seen to be anteriorly translated with respect to the next inferior spinolaminar junction (useful differentiating feature from isthmic spondylolysis). However, these features are not as well-depicted on radiographs as on cross-sectional imaging.

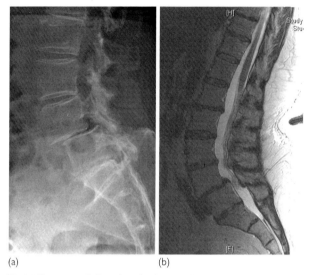

(a)   (b)

Fig. 8.7 Degenerative listhesis. Lateral radiograph (a) shows grade 1 (25%) slip of L4 on L5; (b) the sagittal T2W MRI shows reduction in the calibre of the spinal canal as a result of the degenerative listhesis (c.f. in lytic listhesis the canal is increased in diameter).

Computed tomography (CT)
Demonstrates the above mentioned features to better effect. The degree of facet hypertrophy is better depicted along with its effect on the foramina and spinal canal.

Magnetic resonance imaging (MRI)
The best modality to demonstrate the effects of the facet arthrosis on the neural structures, to assess the degree of spinal stenosis and demonstrate any cysts associated with the arthrosis. There is reduction in the amount of cerebrospinal fluid (CSF) around nerve roots. Hourglass configuration of thecal sac on sagittal imaging and trefoil/triangular appearance on cross-sectional imaging. However, cross-sectional studies are performed usually with the patient in a supine position and therefore not the physiological position that usually reproduces patient symptoms. The calibre of the spinal canal has been shown to vary dynamically in weight bearing erect posture and also during flexion/extension.

Spondylolysis and lytic (isthmic) spondylolisthesis

Although commonly used to describe a defect in the pars interarticularis, the term 'spondylolysis' strictly means a defect/gap in the vertebra, and can occur anywhere in the posterior elements including the pedicle, lamina or facet joint itself.

Incidence: 4–6% of general population.

Aetiology: not established but the general consensus is stress/repeat microtrauma. Hereditary hypoplasia of the pars may be contributory in some cases.

Epidemiology: commonly seen in adolescents and young adults. Associated with certain sports like cricket, gymnastics, diving, football, and hockey. Commonly occurs at the L5 and L4 levels (> 95%) but can rarely occur higher up in the lumbar spine. Bilateral in 75%. More common in boys and white population (Caucasian: Afro-Caribbean—3:1). The typical patient is a young adolescent boy.

Clinical features

Low back pain, exacerbated with sport and relieved after a period of rest. Normal biochemistry. Nerve root compression can occur after spondylolisthesis.

Imaging modalities (Fig. 8.8)

There are two distinct imaging features in these patients which can coexist in the same patient: spondylolysis and stress reaction. CT is the best modality to identify spondylolysis while MRI and bone scan are best to identify the stress related changes.

Radiographs

Radiolucent band at the pars interarticularis +/– sclerotic border. May be associated with spondylolisthesis. Reactive sclerosis and hypertrophy of contralateral pedicle due to stress related changes. On an oblique view the pars defect with surrounding sclerosis resembles the collar of a 'Scottie dog'. The spinal canal in spondylolytic spondylolisthesis is normal or widened (degenerative spondylolisthesis results in spinal canal narrowing).

Computed tomography (CT)

Excellent at demonstrating the pars defect and may show associated contralateral chronic stress changes. CT is also useful to predict healing. Narrow irregular defect with little or no sclerosis—good chance of healing, wide defect with markedly sclerotic margins and hypertrophied fracture ends—poor chance of healing. Serial CTs are also useful to monitor healing and response to treatment. CT should be performed with isometric volume imaging of the lower lumbar spine wherever current multidetector row CT (MDCT) is available. Reverse gantry CT is only indicated where MDCT is not available.

Other imaging modalities

Isotope bone scan

With or without SPECT demonstrates increased activity at the pars. The anatomical information is however poor and may need further imaging to confirm. Stress changes with out spondylolysis also demonstrates similar increased uptake to spondylolysis (false positives). However, the bone scan is very sensitive.

Magnetic resonance imaging (MRI)

Can demonstrate not only the pars defect but also stress changes. However, conventional 2D sequences are not routinely performed in the correct plane to assess pars interarticularis routinely (false negatives). The advent of fast 3D spin echo imaging may change this in the future and MRI may be able to identify both the stress changes and spondylolysis accurately.

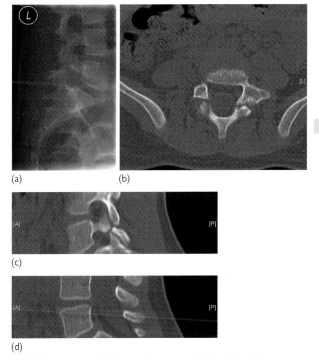

(a) (b)

(c)

(d)

Fig. 8.8 Lateral radiograph (a) shows bilateral spondylolytic defects in the pars interarticularis at the L5 level with spondylolisthesis at the L5/S1 level. Reformatted images from an MDCT examination (b, c, and d) demonstrate the bilateral pars defects and the relative increase in the dimension of the spinal canal compared to degenerative listhesis where there is generally a decrease in spinal canal dimension.

Other causes of spondylolisthesis

Other causes of spondylolisthesis include dysplasia, trauma, iatrogenic, and other pathological conditions.

Dysplastic spondylolisthesis (Fig. 8.9)

This is caused by an abnormality in the orientation of the facet joints in the lumbar spine. Normally, the facets are orientated coronally in the lumbar spine restricting anteroposterior movement. In dysplastic spondylolisthesis the orientation of the facets is either horizontal or sagittal.

Traumatic spondylolisthesis

Usually secondary to severe trauma. Results from fractures or dislocations involving components of the neural arch including the pedicle or facet joint. CT and MRI demonstrate the degree of bone injury and the associated ligamentous injury necessary to cause the slip. The commonest traumatic spondylolisthesis is the 'Hangman's fracture' that occurs in the C2 vertebral body.

Iatrogenic spondylolisthesis

This can follow laminectomy or facetectomy. If posterior decompression surgery is performed on the spine without fusion, there is a 30% incidence of spondylolisthesis.

Pathological spondylolisthesis

This can be caused by any condition that causes a generalized weakening of bone including Paget's disease, osteoporosis, osteogenesis imperfecta, achondroplasia, osteopetrosis. Other pathological processes like tumour and osteomyelitis can cause localized weakening of the posterior elements and result in spondylolysis and spondylolisthesis.

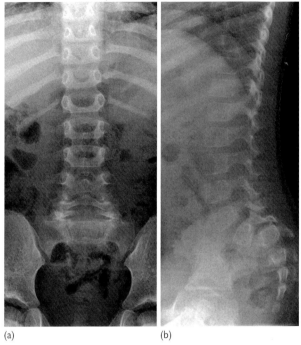

(a)   (b)

Fig. 8.9 Dysplastic spondylolisthesis. AP (a) and lateral (b) radiographs of the lumbar spine demonstrate L5/S1 spondylolisthesis due to hypoplasia of the posterior elements of L5, with a more horizontal orientation of L5 facets facilitating the spondylolisthesis.

Disc infection (pyogenic)

Prevalence: more common in children and >50 years. In adults, it is associated with underlying immunodeficiency and chronic illnesses like HIV, underlying malignancy, renal and other organ failure, malnourishment.

Aetiology: blood-borne invasion is the most common. However, direct inoculation can occur due to surgery, discography, myelography, chemonucleolysis, biopsy, cementoplasty, and other interventional procedures.

Organisms: Staphylococcus Aureus most common. Gram negative organisms in immunocompromised and IV drug users.

Pathogenesis: the disc has intrinsic vascularity in children and infection can start in the disc space. However, in adults, the disc itself is avascular and infection usually starts in the anterior inferior aspect of the vertebral body. The infection then spreads across the disc space to involve the end plate of the adjacent vertebra. Phlegmon or abscess formation in the epidural space can cause cord or neurological compromise either due to direct compression or due to secondary vascular compromise. Direct infection of the cord is rare.

Usually involves the lumbar spine, unusual in the cervical and upper thoracic spine.

Clinical features

Subacute (weeks) history of fever, malaise, back pain, referred pain and occasionally neurological symptoms. Raised erythrocyte sedimentation rate (ESR), CRP which increase progressively.

Imaging modalities

Radiography

Radiographs can take 2–4 weeks after onset of symptoms before early features are evident. Decreased disc height, indistinct and destroyed end plates. End plates become sclerotic later on in illness (healing). Eventually fusion may occur across disc space.

Computed tomography (CT)

Shows the above features and may in addition show adjacent inflammatory soft-tissue mass and epidural inflammatory mass (phlegmon or abscess).

Magnetic resonance imaging (MRI) (Fig. 8.10)

The most sensitive and specific imaging option. Oedema (low T1W and high T2W signal) adjacent to the end plates, destruction of end plates, abnormal signal in the disc compared to adjacent disc (often high signal on T2W), loss of disc height. MRI also demonstrates the surrounding soft-tissue masses. Epidural extension and neurological compression is best demonstrated by MRI. Intravenous gadolinium administration is useful to demonstrate the size and location of abscesses (high signal on T2W, rim enhancement after gadolinium with no central enhancement). Gadolinium enhancement is seen in disc space.

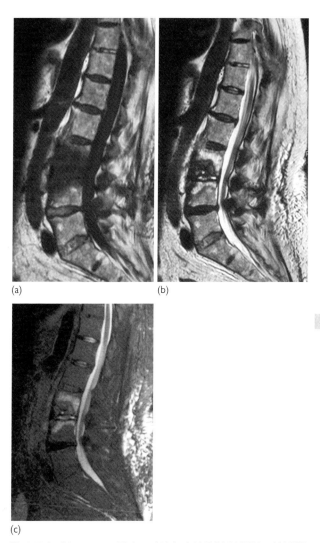

(a)

(b)

(c)

Fig. 8.10 *Staphylococcus* spondylodiscitis L3/4 level. (a) T1W; (b) T2W; and (c) STIR sagittal MRI images demonstrate high signal (fluid) in the disc space on T2 and STIR images. The end plates are irregular and destroyed. There is a low signal on T1W images and high signal on T2W images in the L3 and L4 vertebral bodies in keeping with oedema.

Other imaging modalities
Bone scan detects infection earlier than radiographs, but does not give anatomical information and other imaging is usually necessary afterwards. An MRI is therefore preferred.

Image (fluoroscopic or CT) guided biopsy can help isolate the organism and assess antibiotic sensitivity.

Differential diagnosis
Degenerative disc disease (especially Modic type 1 end plate changes)— vacuum phenomenon is highly specific for degenerative disease. Gas in the disc space is not usually seen in infection. No gadolinium enhancement in disc space.

Tumours do not usually cross disc space. Myeloma can occasionally spread to the adjacent vertebra underneath the anterior longitudinal ligament.

Complications
Neurological compression (needs immediate surgery to relieve compression), kyphosis.

Table 8.1 Differentiating features of pyogenic and tuberculous spondylodiscitis

	Pyogenic	TB
Fever	++	+/−
Toxic	More common	Uncommon
ESR, CRP	Raised	Significantly raised
Immunocompromise, chronic illness	May be present	More common
Multilevel involvement	Uncommon	More common
Abscess formation	Small and few	Large and multiple
Subligamentous spread	Uncommon	More common
Vertebral body involvement with no disc involvement	Less common	More common
Calcification in soft issues	Uncommon	Frequent

Disc infection (non-pyogenic)

Tuberculosis (see Fig. 8.11)

Less common than pyogenic infection, more commonly associated with immunocompromised states.

Prevalence: more common in elderly, ethnic minority groups (Asian, African, and eastern European descent). Has increased in recent years due to human immunodeficiency virus (HIV)-associated disease. Alcoholism and drug addiction are contributory.

Pathogenesis: similar to pyogenic and is usually haematogenous. The degree of destruction may be less with tuberculosis (TB) due to lack of proteolytic enzymes. The infection in these cases can spread beneath the ligamentous structures to involve adjacent vertebrae. It is important to note that during the healing phase there may be continued bone destruction for a few months which should not be misconstrued to be poor response to treatment. Similarly paravertebral abscesses may take many months to completely resolve.

A high degree of suspicion is necessary and the histopathologist and microbiologist should be alerted to the possibility of TB at the time of biopsy. Special culture media may be necessary.

Clinical features

Variable and unreliable. Persistent spinal pain, local tenderness and limitation of mobility. May be afebrile. Neurological deficit (20–40%). Raised ESR (80%). Up to 50% have a normal chest X-ray.

Imaging modalities

Radiologic features

Most commonly involves the thoracolumbar junction. Radiographs are insensitive to early disease. The presence of paraspinal abscess may be apparent by the displacement of paraspinal fat stripe in the thoracic spine and psoas displacement in the lumber spine. Calcification may be seen in the affected paraspinal tissues.

Computed tomography (CT)

CT demonstrates the bone destruction to better effect. Intravenous contrast medium helps in identifying abscesses which are more common and larger in TB than pyogenic infection.

Magnetic resonance imaging (MRI)

The preferred imaging technique.

Although it is impossible in a number of cases to differentiate pyogenic from tuberculous spondylodiscitis, some features are helpful and described in Table 8.1.

Differential diagnosis

Degenerative disc disease as discussed previously. Tumours causing contiguous vertebral involvement like lymphoma, myeloma, and chordoma can be difficult to differentiate. If the disc is not involved it can be difficult to differentiate from metastasis or myeloma.

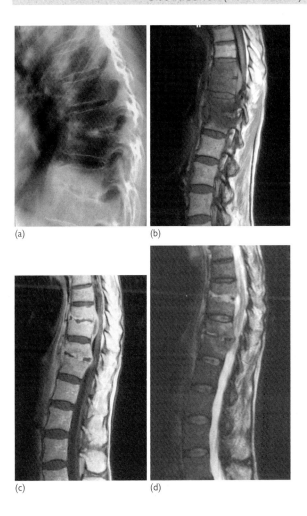

(a) (b) (c) (d)

Fig. 8.11 Tuberculous spondylodiscitis. Lateral radiograph (a) shows endplate destruction, sclerosis, and disc height loss. Pre-contrast T1W (b), post-contrast T1W (c), T2W (d) sagittal images show end plate destruction, multilevel involvement (T9/10 and T11/12), high signal in the disc, and large epidural masses causing cord compression. The epidural masses demonstrate rim enhancement on post-contrast image in keeping with abscess. There is also enhancement in the disc space and endplates.

Principles of spine trauma

Spinal trauma is uncommon, but can be debilitating and cause serious disability. It is therefore important to identify injuries accurately and immediately after injury. The severity of injury is proportional to the forces involved in the injury.

Which patients to image

Careful clinical evaluation is required—pain, torticollis, local tenderness, muscle spasms, asymmetry, limitation of movements are all important clinical findings indicating need for imaging.

What images to perform

Radiography

There is significant debate as to the number of radiographic views in the acute setting. In the cervical spine 3-image series (lateral, anteroposterior and open-mouth) is generally recommended (93% sensitive). A single lateral radiograph will miss 21% of injuries. It is important to make sure the C7/T1 junction is seen well. Otherwise additional projections or CT are necessary. Missed spinal injuries are a result of poor-quality radiographs and errors in interpretation (see Fig. 8.12). Adequate radiographs are difficult to perform in the thoracic spine. Normal initial radiographs do not exclude significant injury (can miss posterior element fractures and hyperflexion injuries). Therefore, delayed imaging is necessary if suspicion for injury persists. Flexion/extension views are controversial(can be false negative due to muscle spasm). Passive flexion/extension views in obtunded patients are not recommended and can be dangerous.

Computed tomography (CT)

Bone detail is best demonstrated by CT which also enables multiplanar assessment of bony injury. Ligaments and soft tissues are well assessed by CT. MRI is best to assess cord, neurological structures and other soft tissues including the disc and ligaments.

SCIWORA (spinal cord injury without radiographic abnormality)

This term is used to represent the significant proportion of patients who do not demonstrate injury on radiographs or CT but have a cord/neurological injury. An MRI scan usually shows cord abnormality in these patients. There are, however, a small group of these patients where even the MRI scan does not show any abnormality. SCIWORA is more common in children than adults. SCIWORA usually presents immediately after injury but in some patients can present after a significant period of time.

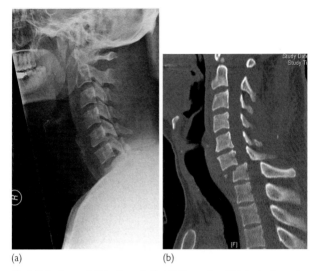

(a)   (b)

Fig. 8.12 Inadequate initial radiograph. On initial inspection, this lateral radiograph (a) appears normal. However, the spine was only seen up to C6 level. Sagittal CT reconstructions (b) shows >50% anterior displacement of C5 over C6 denoting bilateral facet dislocation. *Inadequate radiographs are a major cause for missed injuries.*

Radiographic interpretation

Alignment, Bones, Cartilage and joints, Soft tissues (ABCS).

Alignment is assessed by drawing lines along the anterior vertebral margins, posterior vertebral margins and the spinolaminar junctions which usually form gentle curves (Fig. 8.13). Any sudden steps in these curves should be carefully interrogated. Normal alignment should be seen at the facet joints. The interspinous distance at a particular level should be similar to the level above and below. Radiographic signs of instability include widened interpediculate distance, widened interspinous distance, incongruous facet joints, vertebral displacement, severe vertebral compression (>40%), and disrupted posterior vertebral body margin.

Bones are assessed for any compression or fracture lines. Cartilage includes the disc which should be of the same height as the adjacent discs. The facet and uncovertebral joints should be aligned. The soft tissues are assessed for widening.

Children vs. adults

Spinal injuries are less common in children than in adults. Cervical spine injuries form a larger proportion of the total spinal injuries in children (60–80%) compared to adults (30–40%). The upper cervical spine (up to C3) is particularly liable to injury in young children. The clinical examination can be difficult in young children and a lower threshold of suspicion is necessary. A number of normal variants and ossification centres can be confused with injuries. By the age of 8 years, the pattern of spinal trauma is similar to adults. The vertebral column in children is more elastic than adults and therefore can withstand a higher proportion of forces. However, the spinal cord does not share the same degree of elasticity and therefore SCIWORA is more common in children than adults. The long-term prognosis is better in children because of the capacity of the spine for growth and remodelling.

Classification

Although there are a number of classification systems, there is as yet no perfect classification. They are either over-elaborate and unusable or they are over-simplified and do not include the whole range of possible injuries. The most commonly system is the Denis three-column concept (Fig. 8.14)—the anterior column consists of the anterior two-thirds of the vertebral body, middle column extends to the posterior third of the vertebral body, posterior column extends from the posterior border of vertebral body to the tips of the spinous processes. Involvement of any two contiguous columns infers instability.

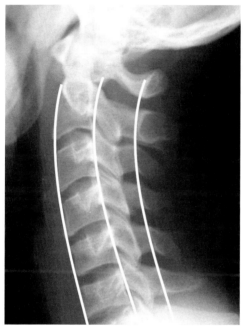

Fig. 8.13 Lines used in assessment of normal spinal alignment.

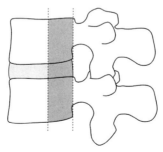

Fig. 8.14 Denis three-column concept. The anterior column comprises the anterior two-thirds of the body, the middle column comprises the posterior third of the vertebral body and the posterior column comprises the posterior elements behind the vertebral body.

Stability
Spinal stability can be described as a condition when there is no risk of increased spinal deformity or neurological deficit over time. There are two broad factors: mechanical stability and neurological stability.

Associated injury (brain, visceral, other spinal)
If one level of injury is seen, there is frequently a further injury in the vertebral column. Using radiographs, this is 15% while with MRI approximately 45% of patients have additional injury in the rest of the vertebral column. Brain injury is frequently associated with cervical spine injury and abdominal visceral injury is associated with lap-belt injury of the thoracolumbar spine.

Sequelae
Cord injury can lead to atrophy, syringomyelia or myelomalacia. Inadequately treated spinal injury may lead to kyphosis, non-union leading to instability, pseudoarthrosis.

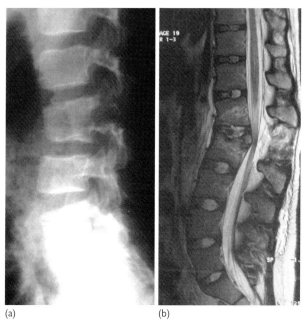

(a)   (b)

Fig. 8.15 Three-column injury. Lateral radiograph (a) and Sagittal T2W MRI (b) show a flexion distraction injury at the L1/L2 level. Flexion anteriorly causes compression of the vertebrae and injury to the disc. Note the soft tissue swelling anteriorly. Distraction posteriorly causes disruption of the interspinous ligaments and widening of the interspinous distance at L1/L2 compared to other levels.

Cervical spine trauma

In young children (<8 years), injuries are more common in the upper cervical spine, from the occiput to the C2/3 level. In older children and adults, injuries more commonly involve the C5–C7 levels. Cord and neurological injury is more common with cervical injuries (40%) than injuries in the rest of the spine (4–0%).

Imaging principles

The initial assessment involves three views (AP, lateral and open-mouth view). Lateral radiograph alone will miss >20% of spinal injuries. The cervical spine cannot therefore be cleared if only a lateral radiograph was preformed.

Most missed injuries are at the craniocervical region and the lowest part of the cervical spine. Therefore, it is important to confirm that all parts of the C-spine are well demonstrated. The open-mouth view can be particularly difficult to perform in children. Pulling the arms down or a Swimmer's view can help to see the C7/T1 level. It is reasonable to extend the CT scan of the head to include the upper cervical spine in all patients with associated head injury. This group of patients are more likely to have spinal injury and less likely to yield good-quality radiographs.

In patients with inadequate radiographs and in those with suspicion of unstable injury, a CT scan should be performed to clearly define injury pattern and facilitate management. The cervical cord is more susceptible to SCIWORA than any other spinal level. MRI scan is necessary in all patients with neurological signs after injury, even if radiographs and CT are normal.

The National Emergency X-Radiography Utilisation Study (NEXUS) low risk criteria and the Canadian cervical spine rules are used in trauma departments to identify patients that need radiographs.

Radiographic assessment

Spinal stability is dependant on both bony and soft-tissue structures. Radiographs only demonstrate bony detail. Soft-tissue injury is implied by the alteration in relationships between bony structures and should be carefully sought. It is also important to realize that the radiographs are performed at rest and may appear innocuous while there might have been significant displacement at the time of injury. Any minor malalignment, angulation, displacement, or abnormal bony relationships should be thoroughly interrogated.

Spinal injuries can be broadly divided by the main direction of force applied at the time of injury (flexion, extension, axial loading, flexion rotation, lateral flexion). The patterns of injury resulting from these forces can be understood using the Denis model of three columns described in the previous section.

Flexion (50–75%): usually, the middle column acts as a fulcrum. In flexion, the anterior column is subjected to compressive force and the posterior column is subjected to distraction/tension. During flexion of the head, maximum forces act between C4 and C7, which is the common site for these injuries.

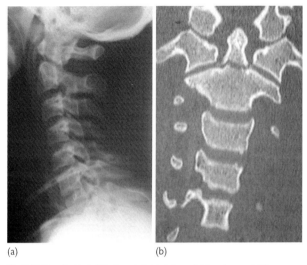

(a) (b)

Fig. 8.16 Type II odontoid fracture. Lateral radiograph (a) and coronal CT reconstruction (b) show a fracture through the base of the odontoid with slight posterior displacement in keeping with an extension injury.

The anterior injury can be seen as a *wedge fracture* or *disc injury* (seen as disc height loss). The posterior distraction injury can cause widened interspinous distance, *spinous process fracture, bilateral facet dislocation*. The combination of anterior and posterior injuries can result in unstable injury with *anterior subluxation*. Some specific types of flexion injuries include:

- *Odontoid fracture*. Odontoid fractures can also occur with extension. The dens displaces anteriorly with flexion and posteriorly with extension. Three types:
  - type I—an oblique fracture limited to dens
  - type II—transverse fracture through the base of the dens (most common—see Fig.8.16)
  - type III—oblique fracture at the base of dens extending into the body of axis.
- *Clay-shoveller's fracture*: avulsion injury of the C7 spinous process.
- *Flexion teardrop fracture*: this is one of the most severe and unstable injuries of the cervical spine. Frequently associated with cord injury. There is comminuted fracture of the vertebral body with a characteristic triangular or quadrangular fragment at the antero–inferior corner. There is also a sagittal split in the body and frequently bilateral fractures of the posterior elements. There may be variable degree of facet dislocation and interspinous widening from ligament injury (Fig. 8.17).

Extension (20–30%): there is compression force on the posterior elements and tensile force at the anterior column. There is prevertebral swelling, widening of the anterior disc space and a variable degree of injury to the posterior elements including fractures of the lamina. There can be a resultant anterior or posterior subluxation. Specific types of extension injuries include:

• *Hangman's fracture:* bilateral neural arch fractures of C2, prevertebral soft-tissue swelling, anterior subluxation of C2 over C3, avulsion of anterior inferior corner of C2 (Fig. 8.18).

• *Extension teardrop fracture:* small avulsion fragment at the anterior inferior corner (see Fig. 8.19).

• *Extension-type odontoid fracture.*

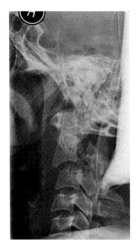

Fig. 8.17 Flexion teardrop fracture. Lateral radiograph shows a large fragment from the anterior inferior aspect of the C4 vertebra. Also note the significant posterior displacement of the remaining vertebral body. There is also increase in the facet joint space at this level compared to the other levels. This is a significant injury and is associates with neurological damage in a large majority of patients.

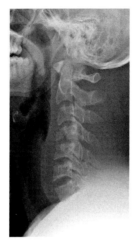

Fig. 8.18 Hangman's fracture. Lateral radiograph demonstrates anterior subluxation of C2 over C3. There isa fracture of the posterior neural arches of C2.

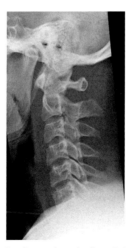

Fig. 8.19 Extension teardrop fracture. Lateral radiograph shows a tiny avulsion fragment at the anterior inferior corner of C3. There is also increase in the prevertebral soft-tissue thickness.

Axial loading: This results from compressive force applied to all three columns of the spine. This causes compression of the whole of the vertebral body. When the degree of compression is excessive, the IVD is driven into the vertebral body which explodes into several fragments and a burst fracture results. Radiographic features include vertebral height loss, encroachment of the spinal canal by displaced bone fragments (usually posterosuperior corner), and disruption of the posterior vertebral body cortical outline. There is variable degree of posterior element fractures and ligament injuries, the presence of which make this fracture potentially unstable.

A specific type of axial injury is the Jefferson's fracture (Fig. 8.20), which is a communited fracture of the C1 ring. There are fractures involving both the anterior arch and the posterior arch of C1. The axial load causes the lateral masses of C1 to displace laterally compared to C2 on the open-mouth view.

Flexion rotation: the ligaments in the spine can withstand reasonable compressive and tensile forces but are particularly susceptible to rotational injury.

A specific type of rotational injury is unilateral facet dislocation. There is less than 25% anterior subluxation of one vertebra over the other (>50% subluxation with bilateral facet dislocation).

Lateral flexion/shearing:
• Transverse process fracture
• Lateral vertebral compression
• Uncinate process fracture

Other specific injuries due to combinations of these forces include:
• *Atlantoaxial instability* (hyperflexion and shearing): this is usually atraumatic and is commonly seen in rheumatoid arthritis, Down's syndrome and is due to transverse ligament rupture. Flexion/extension radiographs may be necessary to diagnose this injury. On the lateral radiograph there is increase (>2.5mm in adults and >5mm in children) in the distance between the anterior cortex of the dens and the posterior cortex of the anterior arch of atlas. Traumatic cases are associated with Jefferson's fracture.

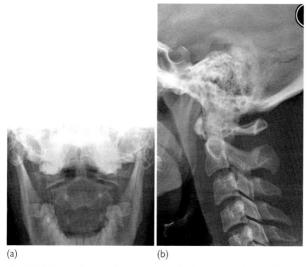

(a)   (b)

Fig. 8.20 Jefferson's fracture. Open mouth view (a) shows the overhanging C1 lateral masses compared to C2 lateral masses due to a burst fracture of C1. This injury is difficult to identify on the lateral radiograph (b) apart from the increased soft-tissue thickening anteriorly.

Cervical spine osteoarthritis

Degenerative changes (OA) affect the discovertebral joints, the apophyseal joints, the uncovertebral joints (also known as neurocentral or joints of Luschka);, and the longitudinal ligaments of the spine. Degenerative changes in the cervical spine are very common with increasing age and somewhat more common in men: they can be seen on radiographs in the majority of people by the age of 50.

OA of the cervical spine is the commonest cause of neck pain and neurological symptoms in adults.

Imaging modalities
Radiography

- Radiographically the disc appears narrowed and a vacuum sign may be seen within it as a linear black area.
- Bony sclerosis is seen at the adjacent margins of the vertebral bodies due to bony eburnation, which may be closely apposed in severe disease.
- Lucent lesions with a surrounding rim of sclerosis may be present adjacent to the vertebral end plates: Schmorl's nodes. They represent nucleus pulposus displaced from the disc.

Spondylosis refers to the development of osteophytes protruding from the superior and inferior margins of the vertebral bodies and are most prominent on the anterior and lateral aspects of the vertebrae (Fig. 8.21). They can be distinguished from the syndesmophytes seen in spondyloarthropathies by the fact that the initial angle of the bony outgrowth is directed in a more horizontal than vertical direction. Osteophytes can restrict movement and when large they can result in dysphagia.

Apophyseal joints

These are synovial joints and as such are subject to osteoarthritis, which affects most often the middle and lower parts of the cervical spine. This is manifest as joint-space narrowing, subchondral sclerosis of bone due to bony eburnation, osteophytosis and can eventually lead to ankylosis. The altered bony structure can lead to weakening of ligaments and segmental instability.

Uncovertebral joint (Fig. 8.22)

With loss of disc height, the uncovertebral joints are pressed closer together and osteophytes form at their margins. Posteriorly these can encroach on the intervertebral foramen and press on cervical nerve roots, giving rise to radicular symptoms in the arms.

Ligaments

The anterior and posterior longitudinal ligaments may become calcified or ossified. The ligamentum flavum may become thickened and kinked and encroach on the spinal canal; in conjunction with posterior osteophytosis and/or disc protrusion at the same spinal level this can result in pressure on the spinal cord and myelopathy.

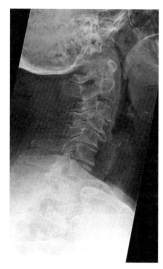

Fig. 8.21 Lateral radiograph shows marked loss of disc heights throughout the cervical spine with large horizontally oriented osteophytes at the C3/4 and the C4/5 levels. There is also degenerative spondylolisthesis at the C3/4 level.

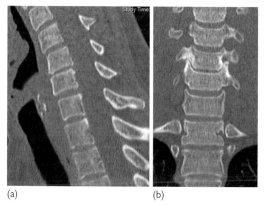

(a)   (b)

Fig. 8.22 Sagittal (a) and coronal (b) CT reconstructions show sclerosis, loss of joint space and osteophytes at the uncovertebral joint at the C5/6 level in keeping with uncovertebral OA. Note the reduced disc height denoting disc degeneration which is always associated with uncovertebral OA.

Cervical spine rheumatoid arthritis

Rheumatoid arthritis (RA) is a chronic immune-mediated inflammatory disorder of unknown aetiology which affects about 0.5% of the adult population and women three times as often as men; it can begin at any age though it is uncommon in childhood. The inflammatory process affects primarily synovial tissue but is associated with damage to adjacent tissues including cartilage, bone, and ligaments. Any part of the cervical spine can be affected although the upper cervical region is involved most commonly.

Clinical features

The cervical spine is involved in most people with RA although this is not always symptomatic. Pain is the most common symptom but nerve root entrapment can cause weakness or paraesthesia in the arms, and cervical myelopathy can result in lower limb weakness, sensory symptoms, ataxia, sphincter disturbances, paraplegia or tetraplegia.

Imaging modalities

The following abnormalities may be seen (Fig. 8.23):

Atlantoaxial subluxation

- Anterior subluxation is most common and results from laxity of the transverse ligament secondary to synovial inflammation. It is defined as an interosseous gap between the back of the atlas and the front of the odontoid peg of >2.5mm (>5mm in children).
- This extent of the gap may not be apparent on lateral views of the cervical spine taken in neutral position so it is vital to request a lateral view with the neck in flexion.
- Extensive synovial inflammatory tissue may be seen at the atlantoaxial level on MRI and erosion of the odontoid peg is common and it may fracture.
- In vertical migration the odontoid peg can enter the foramen magnum and press on the medulla with fatal results. Other forms of subluxation include lateral and, if the odontoid process is severely eroded, posterior subluxation.

Subaxial subluxation

This often affects the mid-cervical region but sometimes there is multilevel subluxation leading to a 'stepladder' appearance on lateral radiographs.

Apophyseal joints

Joint space narrowing, erosion and sclerosis are common and occasionally there is bony ankylosis in long-standing disease. Erosion of spinous processes may be seen.

Disovertebral abnormalities

Disc space narrowing may be seen with irregularity and sclerosis of the vertebral endplates. When this is seen in the absence of osteophytes the picture is typical of rheumatoid involvement, although RA and cervical spondylosis often coexist in older patients.

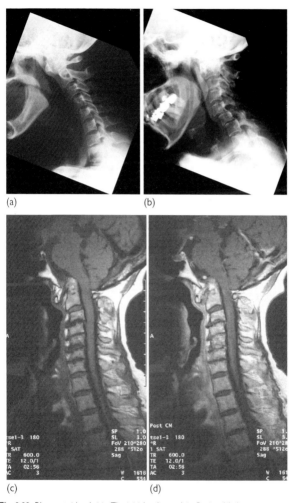

(a) (b)

(c) (d)

Fig. 8.23 Rheumatoid arthritis. The initial radiograph in flexion (a) demonstrates increased atlantoaxial distance in keeping with atlantoaxial subluxation. Radiograph taken a few years later (b) demonstrates subaxial spondylolisthesis at C5/6 and C7/T1 levels. Also note the extensive erosive change at the facet joints. The absence of osteophytes despite the extensive disease differentiates this from osteoarthritis and the absence of syndesmophytes differentiates from seronegative arthropathy. T1W sagittal pre-contrast (c) and post-contrast (d) T1W MRIs demonstrate basilar invagination with superior migration of the dens above the level of the clivus impinging on the medulla. There is enhancing pannus at the subluxed atlantoaxial articulation.

Cervical spine ankylosing spondylitis and other seronegative arthropathies

The clinical and radiological features of spinal ankylosing spondylitis (AS) are similar to other seronegative arthropathies. The differentiating features are discussed elsewhere. AS may occur as an isolated disorder or in association with other inflammatory disorders: psoriasis, ulcerative colitis, Crohn's disease, reactive arthritis, and uveitis.

Pathogenesis

It is a chronic inflammatory disorder of unknown cause which is strongly associated with the Class I major histocompatibility complex (MHC) antigen HLA-B27 and involves cartilaginous and synovial joints as well as the insertions of tendons and ligaments. Although primarily a spinal disorder, peripheral joints are involved in a significant minority of cases. It usually begins in young adult life and has a prevalence of about 1 in 500 of the UK population; men are affected more often than women in a ratio of about 5:1.

Clinical features

People with AS typically experience pain and stiffness of the spine especially at night and early in the morning, or after prolonged sitting during the day. Stiffness of the spine evolves and is associated with a thoracic kyphosis and restricted chest expansion.

Imaging

Discovertebral joints

- Erosions occur at the superior and inferior anterior corners of vertebral bodies ('Romanus lesions') and are associated with reactive sclerosis ('shiny corner'). The erosions in association with new bone proliferation along the anterior surface leading to loss of the normal anterior concavity of the vertebra ('squaring').
- Syndesmophytes (Fig. 8.24) develop with fusion of the bony outgrowths from adjacent vertebral corners. Involvement of multiple vertebral bodies leads to a 'bamboo spine' appearance. In late disease calcification of the disc space is sometimes seen.
- Atlantoaxial subluxation is uncommonly seen in AS.
- MRI can show additional inflammatory and destructive lesions which can be extensive at a stage when there may be only equivocal changes apparent on plain radiographs; changes may be seen in bone marrow or entheses as well as in joints. Focal discovertebral erosions are common and associated 'Schmorl's nodes'. Sometimes the whole vertebral endplate is eroded ('Andersson lesion').

Apophyseal joints

Erosions, subchondral sclerosis, joint-space obliteration and later, ankylosis.

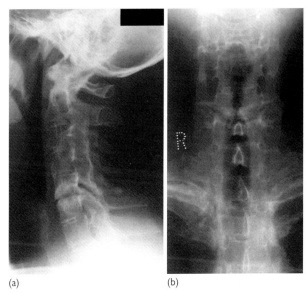

(a)   (b)

Fig. 8.24 AS. Lateral (a) and AP (b) radiographs show fine syndesmophytes through out the cervical spine with fusion across the disc spaces. Fusion is also seen across facet joints. There is a sudden disruption in the flowing ossification at the C5/6 level with sclerosis and irregularity. There is widening of the C5/6 facet joints. Appearances are in keeping with pseudo-arthrosis formation due to 'last unfused segment'.

Fractures

- The ankylosed spine is associated with reduced elasticity of the vertebral column which is more susceptible to fracture than a normal, supple spine.
- Despite the new bone formation, the disease is paradoxically associated with overall reduction in vertebral bone density and osteoporosis, which also increases the risk of fracture.
- Rarely a spinal fracture may be the presenting feature of AS. Depending on the level involved this may result in paraplegia or tetraplegia. The fracture may lead to pseudoarthrosis and segmental instability needing surgery.

Imaging

- Such fractures are often difficult to diagnose on plain radiographs but can be demonstrated with CT or MRI. MRI is the more sensitive and will also show cord deformity and signal and soft-tissue disruption, including rupture of the spinal ligaments, better than CT.

Diffuse idiopathic skeletal hyperostosis (DISH)

DISH is common in older people and is three times more common in men than women. It is associated with increased bone formation at sites where tendons and ligaments are attached to bone in the spine, and also at peripheral sites.

- Diffuse idiopathic skeletal hyperostosis (DISH) is defined as the presence of flowing ossification along the anterolateral aspect of four contiguous vertebrae with relative preservation of intervertebral disc height and in the absence of apophyseal joint fusion or sacroiliitis. In the thoracic and lumbar spine the osteophytes are seen on the anterior and right side of the vertebra. No osteophyte formation is seen on the left side due to aortic pulsation.
- The calcification between four vertebrae distinguishes it from spondylosis and the preservation of disc space from discovertebral degenerative disease, while the lack of apophyseal joint fusion and sacroiliitis distinguishes it from AS and psoriatic spondylitis.
- There is a poor correlation between radiographic evidence of DISH and the presence or severity of symptoms and it is often an asymptomatic finding.
- The anterior aspect of the spine is more affected than the lateral. Bony outgrowths begin at the anterior margins of vertebrae but unlike AS at several millimetres from the discovertebral junction.
- They bridge adjacent vertebrae and further bone is laid down anteriorly so that large bony masses can accrue. The bony outgrowths can become so large that they cause significant dysphagia which may require operative treatment.
- DISH can be associated with ossification of the posterior longitudinal ligament.
- There may be whiskering at the iliac crest, ischial tuberosity, trochanters, and any other enthesis. Osteophytes may be seen at the pubic symphysis and sacroiliac joint (SIJ).
- Enthesitis and ligament ossification can be seen anywhere in the body.

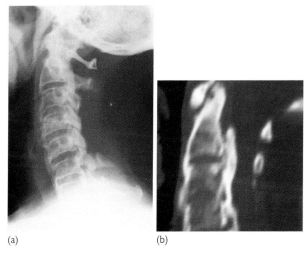

(a)   (b)

Fig. 8.25 DISH. Lateral radiograph (a) of the cervical spine shows extensive flowing anterior ossification separated from the vertebral body by a zone of lucency, throughout the cervical spine. The discs are relatively preserved. Reformatted sagittal CT image (b) shows ossification of the posterior longitudinal ligament. Note the absent posterior elements in the mid-cervical spine. This patient had decompression surgery for spinal cord compression.

Scheuermann's disease

Affects about 4% of the population and is more common in males than females in a ratio of about 2:1. Although the cause is unknown twin studies indicate a significant genetic predisposition. Onset is at puberty.

Clinical features

It often presents in adolescence with thoracic kyphosis whilst pain is a more common presenting feature in adult life. Clinically it has to be distinguished from ankylosing spondylitis although the latter rarely causes pronounced kyphosis in adolescence.

Imaging modalities

Radiography

There is a poor correlation between the presence of radiographic abnormalities and symptoms.

- Scheuermann's disease is defined as anterior wedging of >5° affecting three contiguous thoracic vertebrae.
- It is associated with narrowing and irregularity of the vertebral endplate, Schmorl's nodes (herniation of nucleus pulposus into the vertebral body), vertebral wedging and kyphosis.
- The disc height itself is often narrowed, and there may be reactive sclerosis of the anterior surfaces of adjacent vertebrae.
- Detachment of the anterior apophyseal ring, flattening of the anterior corner of the vertebra, limbus vertebra formation.
- On imaging the presence of sacroiliitis, Romanus lesions or syndesmophytes will distinguish ankylosis spondylitis from Scheuermann's disease.
- The extent of end plate changes can be assessed much more readily by MRI than on plain radiographs.

Treatment

Physiotherapy plus analgesic or sometimes anti-inflammatory medication forms the mainstay of treatment. Spinal bracing can be useful in adolescence. Severe pain or kyphosis may be indications for corrective spinal surgery.

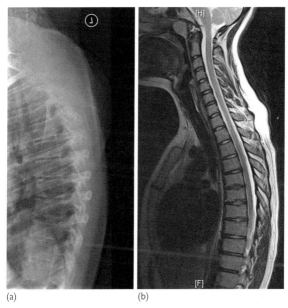

(a)   (b)

Fig. 8.26 Scheurmann's disease. Lateral radiograph (a) and sagittal MRI image (b) demonstrate end plate irregularity involving multiple thoracic vertebrae. There is also minor loss of vertebral height at multiple levels. Features are better demonstrated on MRI than on radiographs.

Sacroiliac joint anatomy

The sacroiliac joint is a large diarthrodial joint, composed of two opposing cartilaginous surfaces. The anterior/inferior third of the joint is a true synovial joint while the rest of the joint is a syndesmosis (formed by interosseous ligament). Recent work has however shown that most of the sacroiliac joint is a symphysis even though the articular surfaces are covered by hyaline cartilage and the bones are held together by strong fibrous tissue.

There is a wide degree of variability with respect to the size, shape, and surface contours. The joint is bounded posteriorly and superiorly by strong ligaments. The anterior sacroiliac ligament is a thinner structure, which is easily ruptured by trauma or joint distension. The posterior capsule is rudimentary and is supplemented by strong ligamentous structures. The main function of the ligaments is to resist motion in all planes. The ligaments become weaker in women during parturition to allow delivery of the foetus.

The nerve supply of the joint is much debated but it is believed that the L4–S3 dorsal rami supply the posterior joint. Some of the confusion surrounding the nerve supply may be due to the close proximity of the SIJ capsule to the retroperitoneum and four nerves; the first two sacral nerves, superior gluteal nerve and the obturator nerve. Therefore, referred pain from the SIJ can be felt in the abdomen, hip, groin, lateral thigh, and even the lower leg.

Extensive networks of muscles support the SI joint and deliver muscular forces to the pelvic bones. Other ligaments such as the sacrotuberous and sacrospinous ligaments help to stabilize the joint. The cartilage on the iliac side of the joint is thinner than the sacral side which accounts for the earlier appearance of erosions and degenerative changes on the iliac side before the sacral side. Age-related changes begin early on the iliac side of the sacroiliac joint during puberty. The iliac surface becomes irregular and rough. These changes progress to form surface irregularities and crevices. These degenerative changes are delayed on the sacral side of the joint. Later on in life, erosions and sclerosis become universal.

The main function of the sacroiliac joints is to provide stability and transmit axial loads to the lower extremities. Although the sacroiliac joint rotates about all 3 axes, the degree of moment is extremely small (a few millimetres of glide and 3° of rotation).

Sacroiliac joint osteoarthritis

Osteoarthritis (OA) of the sacroiliac joint is often seen in radiographs of older people but it is usually difficult to judge its relative contribution to back pain in a given case because most affected people will also have concurrent degenerative changes in the hips, lumbar apophyseal, and discovertebral joints. Sacroiliac joint OA seen on radiographs can however sometimes be confused with mild degrees of sacroiliitis and so could potentially lead to inappropriate treatment.

- SIJ OA is often bilateral but can be unilateral, especially if patients have unilateral hip disease, previous trauma or radiotherapy.
- The subchondral sclerosis is less pronounced than in sacroiliitis and erosion of bone rare, whereas in ankylosing spondylitis extensive irregular erosion is typical.

Imaging modalities

Radiography

As at other sites the radiographic feature of OA of the sacroiliac joints reflect the pathology of OA: joint-space narrowing (loss of cartilage), eburnation of bone (subchondral sclerosis) and osteophyte formation. Subchondral cysts are however, uncommon or small in size.

Computed tomography (CT)

Osteophytes are most common anteriorly at the superior and inferior limits of the joint and can resemble bony ankylosis of the joint on frontal radiographs. However, CT scanning will demonstrate that this appearance is caused by osteophytes overhanging the joint and that although the joint space may be narrowed it is still patent.

Sacroiliac joint ankylosing spondylitis

Sacroiliitis is often the first manifestation of ankylosing spondylitis (AS) and it is extremely unusual for there to be significant involvement elsewhere in the spine in the absence of sacroiliitis, unlike psoriatic spondylitis.

Clinical features

Symptoms can begin in early adolescence but most commonly between the late teens and the fourth decade. Occasionally, the diagnosis is made incidentally on a radiograph taken for other reasons. The typical symptoms are aching and stiffness experienced in the sacroiliac joint region, usually radiating to the buttocks and the back of the thighs.

True radicular symptoms are not features of sacroiliitis and when present suggest a mechanical problem. The symptoms in sacroiliitis differ from those of mechanical back pain in that they are typically worst in bed or after prolonged sitting and are helped by movement and exercise, although vigorous exercise can aggravate pain. The history is particularly important with sacroiliitis as clinical assessment is unreliable, reflected by the poor specificity of the numerous tests which have been proposed.

- In ankylosing spondylitis, sacroiliitis may be unilateral or asymmetric initially but it is usually symmetrical in established disease.
- Both the synovial and the ligamentous portions of the joint are affected but changes are most obvious in the synovial (inferior) part, where changes are more pronounced posteriorly rather than anteriorly, especially in early disease. Entheseal structure, synovium, subchondral bone and bone marrow are all close to each other in this region of the joint.
- The ilium is affected earlier than the sacrum. Initially the margins of the joint appear blurred and then small erosions are visible plus subchondral sclerosis of bone. Gradually new bone is laid down in the joint space and this leads to bony ankylosis. The ligamentous portion of the joint can appear poorly defined and later that too can ossify.

Imaging modalities

Computed tomography (CT)

CT scanning of the sacroiliac joints can be very helpful when radiographic changes are equivocal but involves a significant dose of radiation.

Magnetic resonance imaging (MRI)

- MRI is a sensitive investigation for the detection of early sacroiliitis and will demonstrate oedema of bone on either side of the sacroiliac joint, inflammation in the bone marrow and enthesopathy at the insertions of ligaments. Subchondral enhancement and oedema are seen in active disease while subchondral fatty change in marrow may indicate advanced disease.
- MRI has been used to assess the response to treatment with tumour necrosis factor (TNF)-α inhibitors.

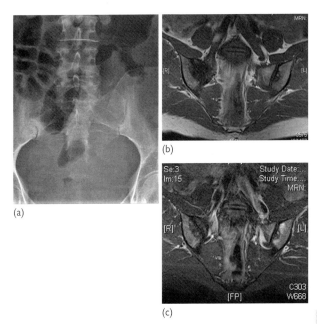

(a)

(b)

(c)

Fig. 8.27 AP radiograph (a) of the SIJ shows bilateral sacroiliitis with erosions, sclerosis and loss of joint space. Features are better depicted on oblique coronal T1W (b) and T2W (c) MR images which demonstrate the erosions on the iliac side with oedema on either side of the SIJ.

Sacroiliac joint psoriasis

Sacroiliitis is seen in about 20% of people with psoriasis and about 40–60% of people with psoriatic arthritis, but there is a poor correlation between symptoms and the presence of abnormalities on imaging. As in the sacroiliitis of AS, erosion of bone and reactive sclerosis are seen, but there tend to be some differences:

- Although sacroiliitis can be bilateral and symmetrical, asymmetrical or unilateral involvement is much more common than in AS.
- The severity of sacroiliitis is generally less pronounced than in ankylosing spondylitis.
- Intra-articular bony bridging is less common than in AS and the sacroiliac joint may remain widened by the erosive process.
- The pelvis often shows enthesopathy with bony proliferation at the sites of attachment of tendons and ligaments such as the iliac crest, ischial tuberosities and pubic rami.

Imaging modalities

Magnetic resonance imaging (MRI)

- MRI is much more sensitive than plain X-rays in showing not only sacroiliitis but also enthesitis at the sites of ligament and tendon attachments. Subchondral bone oedema can be detected in the ilium and sacrum with sacroiliac joint irregularity and erosions during the earlier stages and later periarticular sclerosis and fatty marrow conversion.

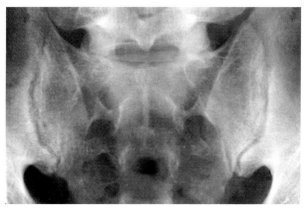

Fig. 8.28 Psoriatic arthropathy. Unilateral sacroiliitis on the right side.

Sacroiliac joint infection

SIJ infection is rare (1–2 cases reported per year). This is therefore a difficult condition to diagnose as it is not commonly suspected early in the disease.

Aetiology: Staphylococcus Aureus is the most common organism. *Brucella Melitensis* infection has been reported in endemic areas. Tuberculosis can also affect the SIJ, although is rare.

Predisposing factors: intravenous drug users, trauma, or any other cause of bacteraemia-like endocarditis.

Clinical features

Unilateral buttock pain, fever, pain on stressing the sacroiliac joint, with tenderness over the sacroiliac joint. Increased ESR.

Imaging modalities

Almost always unilateral disease. Radiographs are insensitive.

Radiography

Radiographs show erosions, widening and destruction of the sacroiliac joint. Bone scan demonstrates increased activity in the involved sacroiliac joint. The bone scan should be performed to include all 3 phases. Infection of the sacroiliac joint is seen as increased uptake in all 3 phases of the bone scan including the early vascular and blood pool phases. Single photon emission tomography (SPECT) images give additional anatomical information.

Computed tomography (CT)

A CT scan will demonstrating the destruction of the sacroiliac joint and any surrounding abscess formation.

Magnetic resonance imaging (MRI)

A MRI scan including STIR images is probably the most sensitive investigation. MRI also demonstrates to better effect surrounding abscess formation.

Differential diagnosis

Unilateral sacroiliac joint involvement with erosions can be seen with seronegative arthropathy. Fever, raised white-cell count, positive blood/joint aspirate cultures, absence of involvement of other joints are features suggestive of infection.

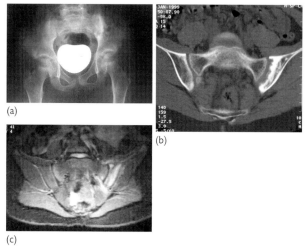

Fig. 8.29 Pyogenic sacroiliitis on the left side. Radiograph (a) shows erosion and destruction of the left sacroiliac joint compared to the normal right side. Axial CT image (b) shows the erosions better. Oblique coronal MRI (c) shows the extensive oedema on the iliac side of the joint. There is also fluid in the joint that distends the capsule and extends into the soft tissues anteriorly, a characteristic feature of infection.

Inflammatory differential diagnosis

Cervical spine

- Cervical spondylosis can usually be distinguished from the inflammatory spondyloarthropathies in that the initial direction of movement of new bone from the vertebral body tends to the horizontal in the former and vertical in the latter, and apophyseal joint fusion does not occur in cervical spondylosis.
- It can sometimes be difficult to distinguish between DISH and inflammatory spondyloarthropathies when bony bridging has developed in the former. However, syndesmophytes in AS typically begin in the region of the annulus fibrosis at the anterosuperior and anteroinferior corners of the vertebral bodies on lateral radiographs, whereas in DISH, the new bone begins from the anterior margin of the vertebral body and a clear space is often visible between the flowing ossification and the vertebral bodies.
- It is usually difficult to distinguish between the different forms of spondyloarthropathies in the cervical spine although in psoriatic spondylitis, syndesmophytes tend to be chunkier than in AS and paravertebral ossification may be seen, although with time such areas fuse with the adjacent vertebral bodies.
- Compared with other parts of the spine the neck is generally affected more severely in psoriatic spondylitis and apophyseal joints are involved as frequently as in AS whereas this is less common elsewhere.
- Spondyloarthropathies can be distinguished from rheumatoid arthritis by the prominence of syndesmophytes and apophyseal joint fusion in the former and of atlantoaxial or subaxial subluxation in the latter.

Thoracolumbar spine

It is often possible to distinguish between the inflammatory spondyloarthropathies in this region.

- Bony bridging is more often symmetrical in ankylosing spondylitis (Fig. 8.30) and that associated with inflammatory bowel disease than in spondylitis, psoriasis or reactive arthritis, in which asymmetry and 'skip lesions' are common.
- In psoriatic arthritis paravertebral ossification and non-marginal syndesmophytes may be present whereas these are uncommon in isolated AS.
- Chunky syndesmophytes suggest psoriatic arthritis.
- As in the cervical spine, the fact that the initial direction of movement of new bone from the vertebral body tends to be horizontal in degenerative arthritis and vertical in spondyloarthropathies helps to distinguish them.
- In long-standing disease DISH can be difficult to distinguish from inflammatory spondyloarthropathies. However, a clear line between the flowing ossification and the fact that bony outgrowths begin from the anterior surface of the vertebral bodies rather than the corners of the vertebrae is typical of DISH.
- Thoracic kyphosis in people with Scheuermann's disease might suggest AS but the absence of syndesmophytes and of apophyseal joint ankylosis in the former distinguishes the two.

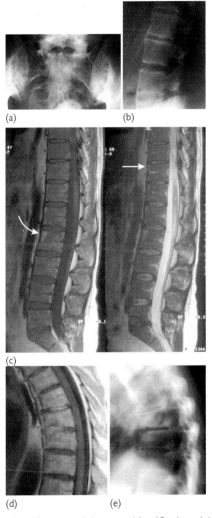

Fig. 8.30 Radiological features in ankylosing spondylitis. AP radiograph (a) shows bilateral sacroiliitis. Lateral radiograph of the lumbar spine (b) shows erosion of the anterior superior corner of the vertebra with a small focus of sclerosis → 'shiny corner' sign or 'Romanus' lesion. Sagittal T1W and T2W MRI sections (c) show high signal at the corners of multiple vertebrae in keeping with Romanus lesions (arrows). Sagittal T1W MRI (d) and lateral radiograph (e) show destruction of endplates, disc height loss and high signal with in the disc in keeping with Andersson lesion.

Imaging modalities

Magnetic resonance imaging (MRI)

MRI is much more sensitive than plain radiographs in demonstrating diagnostic discovertebral lesions in the early stages of AS.

Sacroiliac joints

- Sacroiliitis is more often symmetrical and severe in AS than in psoriatic or reactive arthritis. Bilateral symmetric disease is seen in AS and inflammatory bowel disease while unilateral or asymmetric disease is seen in psoriasis, Reiter's disease, infection and sometimes OA. Sacroiliitis is uncommon in rheumatoid arthritis but when present tends to be asymmetrical with modest erosions, less sclerosis and infrequent ankylosis.
- In hyperparathyroidism, subchondral erosion of the joint can lead to widening of the joint space. There is no joint-space narrowing, sclerosis or ankylosis.
- In psoriatic arthritis interosseous fusion of the sacroiliac joints is less common than in AS.
- Sacroiliitis has to be distinguished from osteitis condensans ilii in which there is symmetrical well-defined triangular sclerosis at the anteroinferior aspect of the iliac side of the joint but the sacroiliac joint space is preserved and there are no changes on the sacral side of the joint; this condition is typically seen in multiparous women.

Imaging modalities

Magnetic resonance imaging (MRI)

- MRI can be used to demonstrate changes in the bone marrow on either side of the sacroiliac joint, and is more sensitive than plain radiographs in showing early erosive change.
- Infection of the sacroiliac joint can be the cause of unilateral sacroiliitis. MRI will show not only erosion and marrow oedema either side of the joint but also fluid within the joint and adjacent soft-tissue fluid collections, sinuses, and fistulae.

Involvement of other areas

- Bilateral symmetrical small joint involvement is often seen in rheumatoid arthritis
- Asymmetrical small joint and entheseal involvement is seen in psoriasis and Reiter's disease. Hand involvement is more commonly seen in psoriasis while feet involvement is more common in Reiter's disease.
- Whilst AS can involve the hips and other large joints, small joints are not typically involved.
- DISH involves the ligament and tendon insertion sites with sparing of the joints themselves. There is ossification at the entheses and of the ligaments.

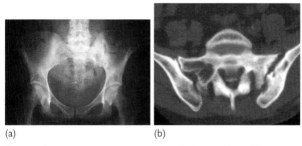

(a) (b)

Fig. 8.31 Post-radiotherapy unilateral sacroiliitis. Radiograph (a) and CT (b) show unilateral left-sided sacroiliitis in this patient with erosions and sclerosis. This patient received previous radiotherapy for a pelvic malignancy.

Table 8.2 Differential diagnostic features of various inflammatory sero-negative spondyloarthropathies

	Ankylosing spondylitis	Inflammatory bowel disease associated spondylo-arthropathy	Psoriasis	Reiter's disease
Sacroiliitis frequency (%)	100	20	40	40–60
Sacroiliitis distribution	Bilateral symmetrical	Bilateral symmetrical	Unilateral or asymmetrical	Unilateral or asymmetrical
Spinal syn-desmophytes	Delicate marginal	Delicate marginal	Bulky non-marginal	Bulky non-marginal
Peripheral arthritis (frequency, distribution)	Unusual, lower limbs	Common, lower limbs	Common, hand	Common, lower limb (feet)
Enthesitis	Common	Unusual	Very common	Very common
Nail changes	None	Clubbing	Onycholysis	Onycholysis
Pulmonary changes	Upper lobe fibrosis	None	None	None

Insufficiency fractures of the sacrum

Insufficiency fractures are caused by normal physiological stress applied to a bone with abnormal elastic resistance or mineralization. Insufficiency fractures of the sacrum are usually seen in elderly women with osteoporosis and often go unrecognized.

Aetiology

Osteoporosis (most common), corticosteroid treatment, osteomalacia, osteopetrosis, osteogenesis imperfecta, Paget's disease, hyperparathyroidism.

Clinical features

The typical history is of fairly sudden onset of severe pain in the lumbar or pelvic region, usually without any history of significant trauma, with localized tenderness and difficulty in weight-bearing. However, the pain may be experienced more diffusely over the lower lumbar or pelvic and buttock region and radiate into the thighs; careful palpation may be required to suggest the precise origin of the pain.

Imaging modalities

Radiography

Insufficiency fractures of the sacrum are rarely visible on plain radiographs, especially as the bones are usually osteopaenic and there may be overlying gas or faecal shadows. The best diagnostic clue on radiographs is the disruption of the sacral arcuate lines with sclerosis paralleling the SIJ. Unless the diagnosis is considered and further imaging arranged then the diagnosis is likely to be missed.

Magnetic resonance imaging (MRI)

Also sensitive and more specific: it will usually show the fracture and surrounding oedema in bone.

Computed tomography (CT)

The most accurate method of demonstrating the sacral fractures and shows the fracture lines, cortical disruption, sclerotic bands, fragmentation, and displacement.

- Both CT and MRI can be used to assess healing of the fracture which can take up to 2–3 years.
- It is not uncommon for insufficiency fractures of the sacrum to be associated with insufficiency fractures elsewhere in the pelvis including the Ilium, supraacetabular region or pubic rami, which will also be seen by these imaging modalities and should be sought.

Other imaging modalities

Isotope scanning

A sensitive method for detecting insufficiency fractures of the sacrum and will typically show an H-shaped ('Honda sign') pattern of increased uptake in the body of the sacrum and sacral alae.

In elderly patients with concurrent malignancy the pain may be wrongly attributed to metastatic disease. Adequate analgesia will usually permit gentle mobilization. Although the pain generally settles over 1–2 months, treatment of the underlying osteoporosis is vital to prevent further fractures.

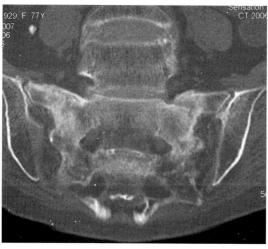

Fig. 8.32 Coronal reformatted CT image shows classic (H-shaped) insufficiency fracture of the sacrum, which has a vertical component that parallels the SIJ on either side and a horizontal component that passes through the body of the sacrum.

Vertebral tumours (primary)

Tumours of the spine can be primary, arising from the structures composing the spinal column, or secondary, due to spread from adjacent or distant structures.

Primary tumours can be benign or malignant. Common benign tumours include haemangioma, osteoblastoma, eosinophilic granuloma, osteochondromas, aneurysmal bone cyst, and giant cell tumours. Primary malignant spinal tumours include chordoma, chondrosarcoma, and osteosarcoma.

Lymphoma and myeloma are variously considered by different authors as either primary or secondary tumours of the spine.

Most malignant tumours (primary and secondary) arise in the vertebral body and extend to involve the pedicles and posterior elements secondarily. Strictly posterior element lesions are far more likely to be benign than malignant.

Clinical features

Pain (85%) and weakness are the most common presentations. Pain can be caused by periosteal stretching, pathological fracture or nerve/cord compression. Pain is progressive and unrelenting unlike mechanical pain. Night pain is common. Pain may be localized to a segment and may be reproduced by percussion of the involved spinal segment.

35–40% present with subjective and objective neurological deficit. Nerve root compression (pain, paraesthesia), cord compression (paraplegia, bowel and bladder dysfunction), cauda equina compression (sphincter dysfunction, saddle anaesthesia). A palpable mass is very rare.

Some tumours (osteoid osteoma) produce painful scoliosis.

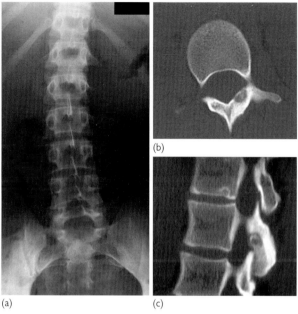

(a) (b) (c)

Fig. 8.33 Osteoid osteoma. Radiograph (a) shows minor scoliosis (painful in this patient) concave to the left centred on the L1 level. Note the sclerosis and the nidus overlying the left L1 pedicle. Axial (b) and sagittal reconstruction (c) CT images show an osteoid osteoma nidus in the lamina and inferior articular process on the left side.

Imaging modalities and characteristics

Osteoid osteoma/osteoblastoma

Scoliosis (lesion at apex of curve on concave side), marked sclerosis (sclerosis minimal if lesion intraarticular), increased uptake on bone scan, MRI shows low signal nidus with marked surrounding oedema, CT best to characterize nidus (Fig. 8.33).

Osteochondroma

Well-defined exophytic lesion (marrow and cortex in the lesion continuous with the vertebra).

Aneurysmal bone cyst

Expansile multiloculated lesion, usually posterior elements with well-defined margins. Fluid–fluid levels on MRI due to blood in the locules.

Haemangioma

Extremely common, usually incidental lesion on MRI of spine (high signal on both T1W and T2W images usually, this can be variable. CT shows 'corduroy' appearance due to thickening of the trabeculae within the lesion. Can extend into the soft tissues.

Eosinophilic granuloma

<30 years, well-defined lucent lesion, vertebral collapse (vertebra plana), can look very aggressive on MRI scan.

Chordoma

Commonly involves sacrum and clivus, can arise from other sites of notochordal rests in the spine (vertebral bodies and nucleus pulposus), starts in the vertebral body and centred in the midline. Expansion and destruction of the vertebra. Low signal on T1W and high signal on T2W images.

Differential diagnosis

Chondrosarcoma, myeloma, metastasis (see Fig. 8.34).

Chondrosarcoma

Rare. Mineralized lesion on radiographs and CT.

Differential diagnosis

The age and position of the lesion are the most important determinants of lesion behaviour. In children benign lesions predominate while in adults over 40 years of age malignant lesions are more likely. Haemangiomata can however be detected at any age but have typical imaging appearances. Biopsy may be necessary.

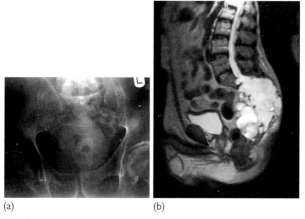

(a) (b)

Fig. 8.34 (a) radiograph shows a large mass overlying the sacrum; (b) Sagittal T2W MRI in the midline shows a large high signal mass centred on the sacrum, a typical appearance for chordoma.

Vertebral tumours (metastases, myeloma)

Metastatic lesions are far more common than primary spinal tumours. Most common primary sites are breast, lung, prostate, and less frequently from renal, thyroid or the gastrointestinal tract.

Myeloma is the most common malignant bone tumour. Commonly involves spine and pelvis. May be solitary (plasmacytoma) or multiple.

Pathophysiology

Haematogenic metastases develop when the tumour cells embolize into the bloodstream, establish in the lungs and then disseminate through the circulation to the rest of the body including the bone marrow. There are therefore lung metastases before development of bone metastases. However, certain tumours can circumvent the lungs through alternative vascular connections with the spinal circulation (prostate via Bateson's venous plexus, lung via segmental artery communications, breast via azygos communications. In adult life, there is conversion of red (haematopoietic) marrow to yellow marrow in most of the skeleton. Red marrow however remains in the vertebral column and pelvis. With its rich network of blood vessels, the red marrow provides a biochemically and haemodynamically suitable environment for metastatic cell deposition and multiplication.

The tumour deposits grow in the vertebrae causing expansion and destruction, extending into the paravertebral soft tissues. This can encroach on the spinal canal and neurological structures (cord, cauda equina, nerve roots) causing neurological symptoms. The involved vertebra is weak and can collapse. This can then lead to spinal instability.

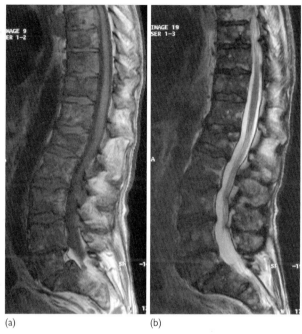

(a)   (b)

Fig. 8.35 Myeloma. Sagittal T1W (a) and T2W (b) MRI images show multiple focal areas of low signal on T1W and high signal on T2W images, one of the patterns of myeloma infiltration.

Imaging modalities
Metastases (see Fig. 8.36)
Imaging choice depends on the degree of clinical suspicion and age. Radiographs, CT and scintigraphy associated with high radiation burden and should be used with caution in young patients. MRI is extremely sensitive and specific but is expensive and not as widely available.

Radiography
Radiographs are insensitive early on in the involvement. Approximately 50% of trabecular bone has to be destroyed before the lesion is detectable on radiographs. Signs include vertebral compression, cortical destruction, paravertebral soft-tissue mass, calcification and the classic 'winking owl' sign (unilateral pedicle destruction). Myeloma classically produces punched-out lucent lesions with multilevel involvement and osteoporosis.

Computed tomography (CT)
More sensitive than radiographs but rarely used for diagnosis (patients not suitable for MRI). Useful for surgical and biopsy planning.

Magnetic resonance imaging (MRI)
The best imaging tool to diagnose spinal tumours, evaluate the effects of the tumour on the neurological structures and differential diagnosis. Superior contrast resolution, no radiation burden, non-invasive and multiplanar capability offer significant advantages compared to other imaging techniques. Low signal T1W, variable signal T2W. Various patterns of involvement—spotty marrow, multiple distinct lesions, solitary lesion or normal signal. May be associated large soft-tissue mass, compression of cord and neurological structures.

Other imaging modalities
Bone scan
Very sensitive to osteoblastic response caused by tumour in surrounding bone seen as foci of increased uptake—'hot spots'. Some tumours (myeloma) with low activity cause 'cold spots'. Not specific and can be positive in trauma, infection, osteoarthritis, mechanical causes and further imaging is often necessary. However, multiple scattered lesions in a patient with known malignancy are virtually diagnostic.

Biopsy
Often necessary to establish diagnosis and to grade the tumour.

Differential diagnosis
Mechanical back pain, disc prolapse, trauma, infection.

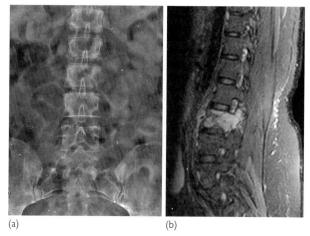

(a)   (b)

Fig. 8.36 Metastases. AP radiograph (a) of the lumbar spine shows destruction of the lateral border of the vertebra and the left pedicle ('winking owl' sign). Sagittal STIR MRI (b) shows the extensive destructive lesion in the L3 vertebra.

Benign vertebral collapse

Vertebral collapse can be of varying degrees ranging from a minor end plate collapse to complete collapse—vertebra plana.

Pathogenesis

Vertebral compression can result either due an excessive compressive force applied to a normal vertebra (trauma) or due to minor force acting on an abnormal vertebra. An abnormal vertebral consistency may be due to insufficient osteoid (osteoporosis), insufficient mineralization (osteomalacia), replacement of bone by abnormal tissue (tumours), normal or excessive bone of poor quality (Paget's disease, osteopetrosis).

The most common cause of vertebral compression in adults is osteoporosis. Vertebral collapse is commonly located in the lumbar and lower thoracic spine.

Aetiology

Trauma, osteoporosis, osteomalacia, osteogenesis imperfecta, sickle cell disease, eosinophilic granuloma, tumour—benign and malignant—infection.

Osteoporosis is commonly seen in postmenopausal women but can be caused by a number of other factors including malnutrition, Cushing's disease, hyperthyroidism, hyperparathyroidism, hypogonadism, diabetes mellitus, acromegaly, renal failure, immobility, rheumatoid arthritis, drugs (steroids, heparin, methotrexate, hypervitaminosis A), radiation therapy.

Clinical features

Pain, kyphosis. Neurological compression may occur with severe degrees of compression. Traumatic or tumour encroachment of the spinal canal or foramina can result in neurological compression.

Imaging modalities

The compressed vertebra can take on various shapes depending on the degree of compression. Anterior compression results in a wedge collapse, central compression causes a 'fish-mouth vertebra' and a generalized compression causes vertebra plana. Schmorl's nodes are seen due to disc herniation into weakened vertebral endplates.

Radiography

Shows diminished density, decreased number and thickness of trabeculae, cortical thinning, and vertical striations (due to marked thinning of transverse trabeculae accentuating the vertical trabeculae).

Computed tomography (CT)

May be necessary to determine the effects of the compression on the spinal canal.

Magnetic resonance imaging (MRI)

Gives the best depiction of effects of compression on neurological structures and further helps to differentiate the various causes of compression.

Treatment

Analgesia in the acute stages, treatment for osteoporosis. If pain is not relieved by simple analgesia, consider bisphosphonate therapy and verte-broplasty/kyphoplasty.

An incidental vertebral collapse seen on a chest radiograph in an elderly patient needs to be regarded as a potential indicator of underlying osteoporosis needing treatment to reduce fracture risk elsewhere.

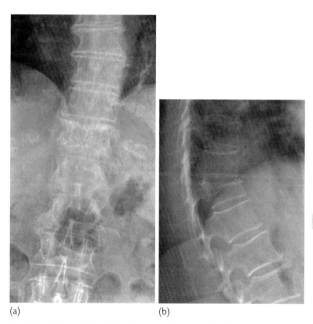

(a)   (b)

Fig. 8.37 AP (a) and lateral (b) radiographs of the thoracic spine show wedge compression of the T12 vertebra. The fracture parallels the superior end plate, a typical feature of osteoporotic fracture. The pedicles are intact.

Differentiating benign collapse from tumour

The differentiation of benign from malignant vertebral compression is clinically necessary to facilitate management. Whilst benign collapses need assessment for metabolic causes, malignant collapses need identification of the exact source as treatment varies greatly with the tumour type.

- Clinically, patients with malignant collapse may have a history of underlying malignancy elsewhere in the body. The typical patient is >40–50 years of age, and may have loss of weight and appetite. These patients are also more likely to have neurological symptoms as the tumour mass may extend into the spinal canal and cause compression. The patient with benign collapse is usually a postmenopausal woman or a patient with underlying metabolic bone disease.
- Patients with benign compressions usually have normal blood parameters other than those expected due to underlying metabolic disease (for example, raised calcium in hyperparathyroidism). Patients with malignant collapse on the other hand have a raised ESR, CRP, and anaemia. There is elevation in the serum alkaline phosphatase due to increased bone turnover. Other markers for malignancy may be positive like prostate specific antigen (PSA), carcinoembryonic antigen (CEA). Patients with myeloma may demonstrate an abnormal globulin in serum or urine (Benz-Jones proteins).
- Osteoporotic collapse usually occurs in the mid to lower thoracic spine. Malignant collapse can occur anywhere in the spine. There may be other extra spinal fractures in osteoporosis in typical locations (wrist, neck of femur, sacrum). Malignant infiltration can occur anywhere but is usually seen in areas with red marrow (in adults, this is the axial skeleton and proximal limbs).
- On radiographs, osteoporotic collapse is usually seen as a wedge or biconcave collapse due to failure of the end plates. Benign collapse is usually limited to the vertebral body with no posterior element involvement. In malignant collapse there may be a variable degree of posterior element destruction. Destruction of the pedicle on one side results in the classic 'winking owl' sign on the AP radiographs. In the thoracic spine, the paravertebral fat stripe may be displaced in malignancy due to a soft-tissue mass.

Imaging modalities

Computed tomography (CT)

CT demonstrates posterior element involvement and any soft tissue mass better than radiographs.

Magnetic resonance imaging (MRI)

MRI is the best imaging investigation to differentiate between benign and malignant compressions. Benign collapses parallel end plates. There may be fluid-filled clefts in the vertebral body paralleling the end plates. The preservation of normal fat signal (high T1W and T2W) in the vertebral body is a useful indicator of benignity. Posterior element involvement and involvement of other vertebrae is seen in malignant collapse.

In malignant lesions, there may be a sizable mass encroaching on the spinal canal causing cord or cauda equina compression. New techniques (diffusion weighted imaging, spectroscopy) are described in the literature but are still not widely used.

- If it is difficult to differentiate benign from malignant lesions even after all the above means, follow-up imaging or a biopsy is necessary.

Table 8.3 Differentiating features between benign and malignant vertebral collapse

	Benign collapse	Malignant
Clinical features	Post menopausal, known osteoporosis. Usually no neurological symptoms unless severe collapse	Known malignancy elsewhere, cachexia. May have significant neurology
Biochemistry	Normal ESR, CRP	Raised ESR, CRP, bone alkaline phosphatase. Other malignant markers PSA, CEA etc.
Spinal level	Commonly mid to lower thoracic spine	Any spinal level may be involved
Radiographs	Collapse parallels disc No paravertebral soft-tissue swelling Posterior elements spared	No pattern to collapse Paravertebral soft-tissue swelling Posterior element involvement (winking owl sign)
CT	No paravertebral swelling Fracture lines seen	Paravertebral soft-tissue involvement
MRI	End plate collapse Fluid cleft Fat preservation in the vertebral body No posterior element involvement No encroachment of spinal canal No paravertebral soft-tissue mass Neurological compression less common	No specific pattern to collapse No fluid clefts Replacement of fat in vertebral body Posterior element involvement Encroachment of spinal canal Paravertberal soft-tissue mass Neurological compression more common

Myelopathy and cord damage

The conus of the spinal cord usually extends down to the level of L1 in adult life, and pressure on the cord at any level above the conus can result in myelopathy.

Aetiology

Trauma, prolapsed intervertebral disc, degenerative disease (spondylosis, thickening of the ligamentum flavum, ossification of the posterior longitudinal ligament), inflammatory arthritis (pressure on the cord from inflammatory pannus), osteoporotic vertebral collapse, tumours, infections: septic discitis or extradural abscess (pyogenic or tuberculous), Paget's disease.

Imaging modalities

Radiography

Plain radiographs may identify lesions such as trauma, tumour, degenerative disease and Paget's disease as the likely pathology but they cannot provide information about the spinal cord.

Computed tomography (CT)

Can demonstrate bone changes well, e.g. the extent of spread of fragments from a burst vertebral fracture or of bony destruction from a tumour, but again it will provide only limited information about the spinal cord.

Magnetic resonance imaging (MRI)

MRI will show not only the relation of the spinal cord to surrounding structures but also the signal from the cord; an abnormal (high T2W) signal will indicate the site at which pressure on the cord is likely to be having an adverse effect on neurological function.

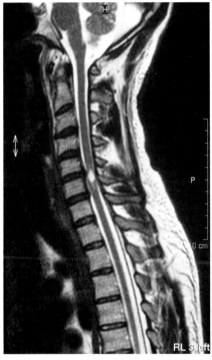

Fig. 8.38 Sagittal T2W MRI shows cervical cord compression at the C5/6 level by a small disc bulge and thickened ossified posterior longitudinal ligament. High signal intensity focus is seen in the centre of the cord in keeping with myelopathy.

Cauda equina syndrome

Cauda equina syndrome is regarded as an orthopaedic or neurosurgical emergency because neurological damage is likely to be permanent unless the pressure on the cauda equina is relieved rapidly. Caused by pressure on the cauda equina, it necessarily indicates a lesion below the level of the conus (usually L1).

Aetiology

Trauma (burst fracture), prolapsed intervertebral disc, spondylolisthesis and degenerative disease: apophyseal joint osteoarthritis +/– thickening of the ligamentum flavum (causing spinal stenosis), tumours, Paget's disease, infection including tuberculosis, arachnoiditis, arachnoid diverticula associated with long-standing ankylosing spondylitis.

Clinical features

Sphincter disturbances are common as is 'saddle anaesthesia': impaired sensation over the saddle region of the perineum, buttocks and back of thighs. Sphincter disturbance usually leads to urinary retention, but dribbling incontinence of urine may occur; there is commonly a lack of awareness of when voiding is required. Constipation is usual but incontinence occurs sometimes. Impotence, diminished reflexes, reduced sensation in lower lumbar and sacral dermatomes. Motor involvement leads to flaccid weakness and wasting of the legs. Pain may be experienced in the sacral or lumbar region. Whether cauda equina syndrome begins acutely (e.g. after trauma) or more gradually depends on the nature of the underlying pathology. A more gradual onset is at risk of going unrecognized and it is important to consider the possibility in anyone with symptoms of sphincter disturbance and check sensation in the saddle area.

Imaging modalities

Magnetic resonance imaging (MRI)

Whilst radiographs may show the underlying cause of the syndrome, the thecal sac and contained neurological structures are only demonstrated non-invasively on MRI scan, which is the imaging investigation of choice. MRI should always be performed immediately when cauda equina compression is suspected clinically and demonstrates the cause, degree, level of compression and aids surgical planning. The T2W images demonstrate complete obliteration of CSF at the affected level. If patient is not suitable for an MRI scan, a CT myelogram can give similar information, but is invasive.

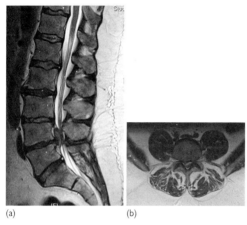

(a)   (b)

Fig. 8.39 Cauda equina compression. sagittal T2W (a) and axial T2W (b) MRI show a large disc sequestration at the L4/5 level obliterating the spinal canal and causing cauda equina compression.

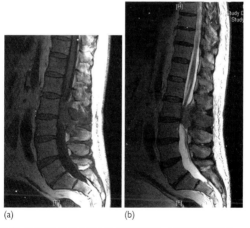

(a)   (b)

Fig. 8.40 Cauda equina compression. Sagittal T1W (a) and T2W (b) MRI show destruction of the L2 spinous process with a large soft-tissue mass from prostate cancer metastasis invading the spinal canal and causing cauda equina compression. Also note further lesions in the T12 and L1 vertebrae in keeping with further metastases.

Syringomyelia

Syringomyelia is the term applied to a cavity within the spinal cord extending over several vertebral segments which may develop as a complication of trauma or as an idiopathic phenomenon.

Pathogenesis

Subarachnoid adhesions (after trauma, surgery, infection, and subarachnoid haemorrhage), disc prolapse or tumours cause obstruction to CSF flow between subarachnoid space and central canal and lead to syrinx formation.

- Post-traumatic syringomyelia is an uncommon complication of spinal cord injury (3%) which may present within a few weeks of injury but may not develop for several years.
- Idiopathic syringomyelia is uncommon, occurring in about 5 per 100,000 population and its causation is unknown. It usually presents in young adult life and the sex incidence is approximately equal.

Clinical features

Because it involves the central part of the spinal cord the crossed spinothalamic tracts are typically damaged early, with consequent impairment of pain and temperature sensation in the hands, and damage to anterior horn cells and corticospinal tracts is also prominent. As the syrinx expands in both horizontal and vertical planes so the extent of sensory impairment in the upper limbs increases and long tract signs develop in the lower limbs. The syrinx may extend into the medulla and be associated with herniation of cerebellar tissue into the cervical canal: Chiari malformation. Syringomyelia is often associated with scoliosis and about 25% of people with syringomyelia develop neuropathic arthropathy (Charcot's joint) particularly of shoulder, but sometimes of elbow, wrist or fingers and much less frequently in the lower limbs.

Syringomyelia may lead to erosion of the posterior surfaces of the vertebral bodies leading to widening of the spinal canal: pathological widening of the canal is present when the width of the canal is 6mm or more than that of the vertebral body.

Imaging modalities

Magnetic resonance imaging (MRI)

The syrinx is not visible on radiographs but can be demonstrated readily on MRI, and syringomyelia is diagnosed more frequently now that access to MRI scanning has become readily available.

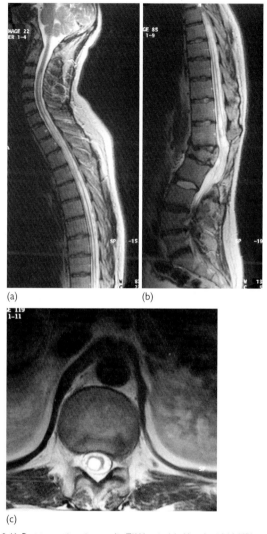

(a)   (b)

(c)

Fig. 8.41 Post-traumatic syringomyelia. T2W sagittal (a, b) and axial (c) MRI demonstrate a syrinx extending from the C3 level to the conus following a previous fracture at the L1 level. The signal in the syrinx is similar to cerebrospinal fluid.

Part 2

Investigations in specific musculoskeletal disorders

Chapter 9

Investigating the child with joint problems

Practical aspects of imaging children

Much of the imaging techniques used to image children are the same as those used in adults but it should be remembered that 'Children are not little adults'—imaging depends on age, clinical condition, and clinical problem.

- Children in the hospital environment are likely to be frightened and distressed. To gain the most from radiological investigations it is important to make the child feel as secure as possible to gain their co-operation and help them relax. Skilled radiography staff experienced in imaging children are invaluable.
- If possible the parents of the infant or child should interact and reassure the child during the study.
- Age-appropriate distractions are invaluable (Fig. 9.1).
- For all children the temperature of the room must be correct to allow them to relax but also prevent hypothermia during long procedures.
- Play therapy can be extremely useful in helping children cope with their fear of an imaging procedure. This may involve the child visiting the hospital several times to become familiar with the radiology department prior to the procedure.
- General anaesthetic (GA) may be necessary. Each case must be considered individually. MRI scans in those under 5 years are likely to require a GA. Plain film imaging and ultrasound should never need a GA and GA should be rarely needed in CT or nuclear medicine (NM) imaging. Sedation can be used but still requires appropriate monitoring by trained staff.

Imaging modalities

In the acute situation plain radiographs, ultrasound and computed tomography are most often used for investigation of musculoskeletal conditions.

Radiography

Trauma is the most common musculoskeletal complaint in children and plain films are the mainstay of radiological investigation. Radiographs, particularly peripheral images, are low dose and easily available. They are also useful for first line of investigation and for follow-up of more complex disease processes.

Ultrasound (US)

Useful for imaging the soft tissues of the musculoskeletal system, e.g. joint effusions, synovial thickening, muscles, and tendons.

Computed tomography (CT)

Involves significantly more radiation than plain films, can be useful in assessing more complex trauma and in the investigation of other bony abnormalities.

Magnetic resonance imaging (MRI)

Difficult to use in the acute situation, but has a major role to play in investigating both soft tissue and bony pathology.

Nuclear medicine

Nuclear medicine must be a planned procedure but still has a role to play in the investigation of musculoskeletal disorders in children, in particular investigation of possible osteomyelitis.

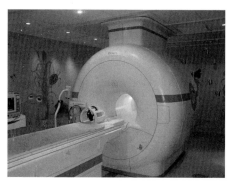

Fig. 9.1 The paediatric MRI at Alder Hey Children's Hospital, Liverpool, UK.

Anatomy of the growing bone

Knowledge of the structure of children's bones and their growth is essential in interpreting paediatric radiographs.

Types of bone

- Tubular bones, found in the limbs.
  - Long bone, e.g. femur—central diaphysis, with a metaphysis, growth plate and an epiphysis at either end.
  - Short tubular bone, e.g. metacarpals—diaphysis and a single metaphysis, epiphysis and growth plate at one end.
- Short bones, e.g. carpal bones in the wrist and metacarpals in the ankle. Initially cartilaginous then ossify from centres during growth to a cancellous (trabecular) centre and hard compact shell.
- Flat bones such as those seen in the skull vault, scapula, and pelvis. Consist of two compact bone layers around a spongy central bone.
- Irregular bones—do not fit into the categories above, e.g. vertebral bodies and facial bones.
- Sesamoid bones which occur in tendons.

Detailed structure of a long bone (Fig. 9.2)

Diaphysis

The shaft of a long bone. Tubular structure with a central medullary cavity containing marrow and a tubular outer cortex of hard compact (lamellar) bone. The cortex contains a network of blood vessels contained in Haversian canals. In children Haversian canals have a simple structure and the bone mineralization is relatively reduced compared to adults. This allows for the 'plastic' bending fractures seen in children (Fig. 9.3). Growth of the diaphysis is by membranous periosteal ossification (↑ width) and conversion of woven bone from metaphysis to lamellar bone (↑ length).

Metaphysis

Lies between the physis and the diaphysis, is flared and wider than the diaphysis.

- Primary spongiosa of the metaphysis lies next to the physis and is formed by endochondral ossification.
- Secondary spongiosa caps the diaphysis and is formed by remodelling of the primary spongiosa. The metaphyseal cortex is perforated by vascular channels and is thinner than diaphysial cortex. With longitudinal growth the metaphyseal cortex becomes thicker and contains less vascular perforations.

Physis (growth plate)

The physis consists of four zones which are largely responsible for the longitudinal growth of the long bones. Fractures extending into the germinal or proliferative zone can interrupt growth resulting in potential deformity.

- Germinal—next to epiphysis contains chondrocyte stem cells.
- Proliferative—dividing chondrocytes in a collagen matrix.
- Hypertrophic—growing cells and collagen matrix. The weakest zone and most often traversed by fractures does not result in arrest of growth.
- Provisional calcification—next to metaphysis. Cells degenerate and collagen calcifies.

Epiphysis

The epiphysis forms the ends of and provides the joint surface of long bones. Initially formed from cartilage which ossifies from a central ossification centre and lined on the joint side by joint cartilage. Contributes to longitudinal bone growth and eventually fuses to the metaphysis when growth is complete.

Apophysis

Lies away from the epiphysis and physis and are initially formed from cartilage but ossifies by secondary ossification. Usually occur at the site of insertion of muscle tendons. Do not have joint surfaces or contribute to longitudinal bone growth.

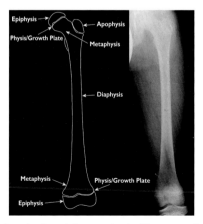

Fig. 9.2 Drawing and radiograph demonstrating the different parts of a long bone.

Fractures in children

Fractures are common injuries in children but each fracture should be considered in light of knowledge of anatomy of the growing child and that visible fractures in ossified bone indicate possible injury in the adjacent cartilage and soft tissues.

Consideration should always be given to normal variants which in children are numerous and can vary with age.

A guide to interpreting plain radiographs

Careful history and examination is always important but in children, depending on the age, the history can be non-specific. For example infants and young children can present with disuse of a limb and careful examination is needed to determine the best sites for, and technique for imaging. The history may elucidate whether disuse is due to injury at all or for example an inflammatory or infective cause. Thought must always be applied to the history of any injury and its clinical and radiological appearances if non-accidental injury of a child is to be recognized.

First line investigation of any fracture should be plain radiographs preferable in perpendicular planes. CT can be a useful adjunct in some situations, particularly in fractures involving large joints such as the knee and ankle.

Assessment of the plain radiograph should be in a number of stages:
- Soft tissue plane—swelling of the soft tissues around a bone or joint is always a useful guide to the site of an injury and can add weight to a diagnosis of a fracture if there is doubt.
- If the injury involves a joint then a joint effusion can also be a useful sign of a fracture. Effusions at the elbow, ankle, and knee are particularly useful signs of abnormality in a joint (Fig. 9.4).
- Fractures in children can be extremely variable from a subtle lucency in the tibia (toddler's fracture—see below Fig. 9.5) to complete dislocation and non-alignment of fracture fragments. In general the outer cortex of the long bone should be smooth and subtle kinks in the cortex can reveal a fracture. An abnormal trabecular pattern with increased density or lucency can also reveal a fracture site. Consideration to underlying lesions, such as simple or aneurysmal bone cysts, causing a pathological fracture should also be given.
- Alignment and stability of a fracture and joint should always be considered remembering that soft-tissue structures such as tendons and ligaments can be disrupted by the same force that caused the fracture. Although fractures in children normally heal easily rotation deformities do not correct themselves.
- Repeat films can be performed if there is any doubt whether a fracture is present or not. Films repeated after 7–10 days will show periosteal reaction and increased bony density at a fracture site.

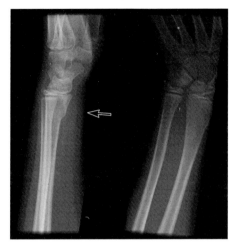

Fig. 9.3 Plain radiograph of the forearm of a child with a greenstick fracture of the distal radius. Note the buckling of the palmar aspect of the distal radial metaphysis without apparent abnormality on the volar side.

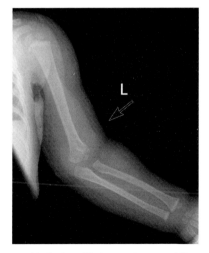

Fig. 9.4 A supracondylar fracture of the humerus in a young child.

Types of fracture in children

The nature of developing growing bones gives them a propensity to fractures not seen in adults.

Fractures of the diaphysis

Fractures of the upper limb, particularly the radius, are most common in children after infancy.

- Classical transverse, oblique, and spiral fractures of the diaphysis can be seen in children as in adults. In children these fractures can be incomplete due to the plastic nature of the bones. Comminuted fractures are not often seen in young children but are more common with increasing age.
- Greenstick involves bending of the diaphysis such that on the convex side of the diaphysis. There is disruption of the cortex and periosteum but on the concave side although there may be micro fractures the cortex and periosteum remain intact.
- Torus/buckle fractures are seen as bumps or kinks in the cortex most often seen in the metadiaphyseal region on the concave side of an injury (Fig. 9.6).
- Plastic/bowing injuries seen as bowing of the diaphysis with no visible fracture seen on plain radiographs but with micro fractures of the bone.

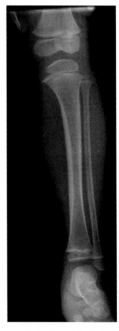

Fig. 9.5 A subtle spiral lucency in the distal tibia of a toddler represents a classic appearance of a toddler's fracture.

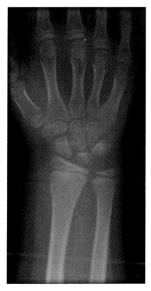

Fig. 9.6 A torus fracture of the distal radial metaphysis. Notice the buckling of the cortex with subtle disruption of the trabeculae.

Fractures of the metaphysis, physis and epiphysis

The growth plate means that fractures around the ends of long bones have a special significance in children. The Salter–Harris classification is used to describe the injury and also implies the possible outcome of such injuries.

Type 1

Separation of the epiphysis across the physis normally occurs through the hypertrophic zone leaving the important germinal and proliferative layers intact. The periosteum of the bone also remains intact and can limit displacement. Type 1 injuries can be difficult to diagnose if there is no displacement and soft-tissue swelling may be the only sign.

Type 2

Involve the hypertrophic zone of the growth plate but then extend through the metaphysis and account for up to 80% of physeal fractures. Usually growth is undisturbed unless there has been an element of compression of the physis.

Type 3

The fracture extends from the hypertrophic zone of the physis through the epiphysis to the joint surface. The germinal and proliferative zones of the growth plate are disrupted but as these fractures are usually in older children and related to partial fusion of the epiphysis growth disturbance is less common. Consideration of further imaging to ensure alignment of the joint surface of the separate fragments should be made.

Type 4

The fracture line extends through the metaphysis, physis and epiphysis to the joint surface. All zones of the physis are disturbed and the potential for tethering of a portion of the growth plate resulting in angular deformation is great (Figs 9.8, 9.9).

Type 5

Rare but involve compression of the growth plate crushing part of the physis and resulting in loss of growth in this area and deformity. These fractures are difficult to diagnose as changes in the height of the physis can be subtle.

Stress fractures

Stress fractures can occur in healthy children, usually as a result of repetitive stress, and as such are usually seen in older children participating in sports.

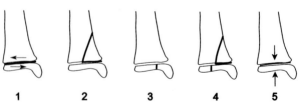

1　　**2**　　**3**　　**4**　　**5**

Fig. 9.7 The Salter–Harris fracture classification of metaphyseal and epiphyseal fractures types 1 to 5.

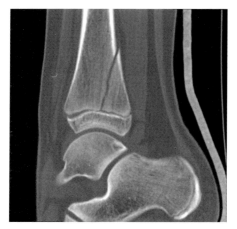

Fig. 9.8 Metaphyseal fracture sagittal reformat.

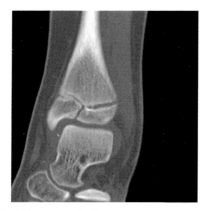

Fig. 9.9 Epiphyseal fracture coronal reformat.

Differential diagnosis of arthritis

Introduction

Joint symptoms in children are common and frequently the result of minor and innocent trauma *but* may be associated with a multiple acute and chronic pathologies, including non-accidental abuse.

Joint symptoms may be associated with potentially life-threatening disorders. As such joint symptoms demand respect from attending healthcare professionals, and require careful assessment by history, clinical examination, and judicious use of radiological imaging and laboratory investigation.

The differential diagnosis of arthritis in children is considerable. We encourage readers to bear in mind the broad range of aetiologies shown in Table 9.1.

Interpretation of imaging findings must *always* be in the clinical context of the child, and is facilitated by close collaboration between clinician and radiologist.

Clinical features

Inflammatory joint symptoms are exacerbated by rest and improve with exercise.

Pain is a typical feature of inflammatory disease, but it must be remembered that younger children do not always verbalize pain as a symptom.

A detailed review of systems is mandatory when assessing the child with joint symptoms: non-specific symptoms such as fatigue, anorexia, weight loss, fever, disturbed sleeping, limping and 'gelling' (stiffness after periods of inactivity) should be sought.

On examination, arthritis is manifest by joint swelling. In juvenile idiopathic arthritis signs may be subtle and it is not unusual for the careful examiner to detect signs in joints not reported as symptomatic by children and carers. Local warmth, limited range of movement, muscle loss and limb length discrepancy are other relevant signs.

Arthritis must be distinguished from arthralgia, as there will be a different if overlapping differential diagnosis to be considered in the child with arthralgia.

A simple system such as 'look, feel, move' may aid the reader when examining joints.

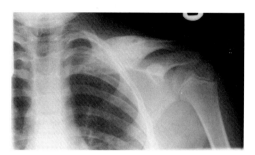

Fig. 9.10 Plain radiograph of the left clavicle showing marked sclerosis and expansion of the mid portion of the clavicle typical of SAPHO syndrome.

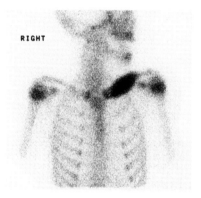

Fig. 9.11 Bone scan of the same patient demonstrating marked uptake in the expanded sclerotic left clavicle.

Septic arthritis

A septic joint will exhibit the classical features of inflammation. An affected hip is often held in flexion and external rotation for comfort; a knee in flexion. All passive movement will be resisted. The hip warrants specific consideration, as increased intracapsular pressure arising from septic arthritis may interrupt blood supply and lead to avascular necrosis of the femoral head, making surgical decompression mandatory in suspected cases.

Fever, malaise, and anorexia are usually seen, and progression of symptoms is often rapid. In neonates features may be non-specific. Children with immunodeficiency states should be evaluated with great care, including those on systemic corticosteroid therapy, as clinical signs of inflammation may be subtle and/or masked.

Imaging modalities

Radiography

Remains the *primary* initial imaging modality for suspected skeletal infections.

In osteomyelitis soft-tissue swelling and a periosteal reaction may be seen within a few days. Bony changes develop later (Figs 9.12, 9.15).

In septic arthritis the early features are osteopenia of the epiphysis, increased joint space and soft-tissue swelling. Later in the disease destructive changes may be seen.

Ultrasound (US)

A rapidly available and sensitive method for detecting joint effusions, especially in the hip. However, it must be emphasized that ultrasound will *not* determine the cause of the effusion.

Magnetic resonance imaging (MRI)

MRI plays a particular role because of excellent delineation of anatomy including soft tissues and bone. T1 weighted fat-suppressed post-contrast images are recommended in both osteomyelitis and septic arthritis.

Other imaging modalities

Radionuclide bone imaging

Sensitive at detecting areas of increased uptake, and may reveal multiple foci within the skeleton. However, the specificity of this method is low and the features may not distinguish septic from non-septic inflammatory lesions (Fig. 9.10).

Malignant disease

Malignant disease should be considered in any child with musculoskeletal pain, especially if nocturnal symptoms present. Peripheral blood films do not always reveal evidence of haematological malignancy.

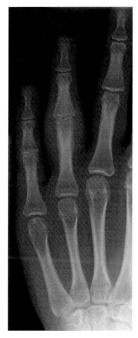

Fig. 9.12 Osteomyelitis. Soft-tissue swelling around the distal portion of the proximal phalanx of the left ring finger. There is also periosteal reaction along the shaft of the proximal phalanx.

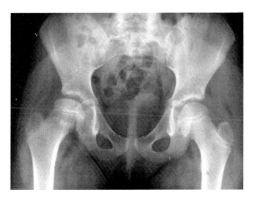

Fig. 9.13 Sclerosis and subchondral lucency of the right upper capital femoral epiphysis in Perthe's disease.

Table 9.1 Differential diagnosis to be considered in the child with arthritis

Aetiology	Relevant condition(s)
Infection	Acute septic arthritis
	Reactive/post-infective arthritis
Idiopathic	Juvenile idiopathic arthritis
Connective tissue disorders	Arthritis associated with inflammatory bowel disease
	Systemic lupus erythematosus
	Juvenile dermatomyositis
	Systemic vasculitis
	Henoch–Schönlein purpura
	Sarcoidosis
Malignancy	Leukaemia (Fig. 9.14)
	Neuroblastoma
Haematological	Sickle cell anaemia
	Haemophilia
Genetic disorders	Cystic fibrosis
	Velocardial facial syndrome
	CINCA syndrome
	Down's syndrome
Drug reactions	
Trauma including non-accidental injury	
Orthopaedic conditions	Perthe's disease (Fig. 9.13)
	Slipped upper femoral epiphyis

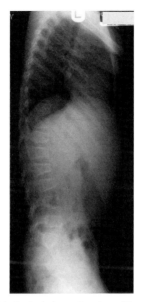

Fig. 9.14 A child with back pain. An impression of overall loss of bone mass with multiple wedge fractures on a lateral thoracolumbar spine. Further investigation revealed a diagnosis of leukaemia.

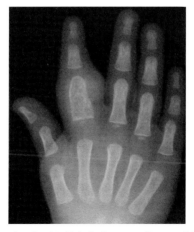

Fig. 9.15 Tuberculous dactylitis. Marked soft-tissue swelling around the base of the right index finger with expansion of the proximal phalanx and irregular destruction of the trabeculae with no periosteal reaction.

Juvenile idiopathic arthritis

Introduction

Juvenile idiopathic arthritis (JIA) is the descriptive term for a group of heterogeneous conditions characterized by *persistent synovitis* of 6 weeks duration, presenting before the age of 16 years, for which no explanation can be found (Petty *et al.* 2004).

Table 9.2 JIA subtypes and associated clinical features

JIA subtype	Clinical features	Red flags/risks
Oligoarthritis:	Persistent Arthritis of 4 or fewer joints within the 1st 6 months Affecting not more than 4 joints throughout the disease process. Frequently children below the age of 5 years Extended Affecting more than 4 joints after the 1st 6 months	High risk of associated uveitis, especially if ANA positive Leg length discrepancy (overgrowth of affected limb)
Polyarthritis RF positive RF negative	Arthritis of 5 or more joints within the 1st 6 months. Subdivided according to presence of RF	RF positive disease rare but equivalent to 'adult' RA
Systemic arthritis	Arthritis with or preceded by daily ('quotidian') fever for at least 3 days, accompanied by one or more of: • evanescent erythematous rash, lymphadenopathy • hepatomegaly and/or splenomegaly • serositis	Arthritis may not be present early in course Mandatory exclusion of infective and malignant conditions
Psoriatic arthritis	Arthritis and psoriasis *or* arthritis with at least 2 of: • dactylitis • nail pitting or onycholysis • psoriasis in 1st-degree relative	
Enthesitis-related arthritis	Arthritis and enthesitis *or* Arthritis or enthesitis with 2 of: • SI joint tenderness or inflammatory lumbo-sacral pain • HLA B27 antigen • onset after age 6 years in a male • acute (symptomatic) anterior uveitis, history of HLA B27-associated disease in a 1st-degree relative	
Undifferentiated arthritis	Arthritis that fulfils criteria in no *or* more than two of the above categories	

ANA, antinuclear antibody; RF, rheumatoid factor; RA, rheumatoid arthritis; SI, sacroiliac.

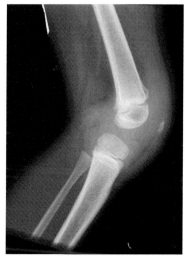

Fig. 9.16 JIA of the knee on a lateral radiograph. Marked soft tissue swelling around the knee with fluid in the supra patella bursa and loss of definition of Hoffa's fat pad (normally seen as a triangle of lucent fat behind the patella tendon).

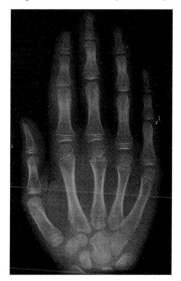

Fig. 9.17 Soft-tissue swelling around the proximal index finger in JIA. Compare to the images of osteomyelitis and TB dactylitis.

Imaging of juvenile idiopathic arthritis

Imaging may facilitate management of JIA at various stages
- To aid the diagnosis—by exclusion of other musculoskeletal disorders, e.g. skeletal dysplasia.
- To define joint damage
- To demonstrate pathology in joints difficult to assess clinically eg hip, shoulder and subtalar joint

Imaging modalities

Radiography

Soft-tissue swelling
- May be only sign in early disease (Fig. 9.16, 9.17)
- Joint effusions are most readily seen in large joints such as the knee

Periarticular osteopenia
- Frequently reported as a sign in 'early' JIA—thought to be a consequence of periarticular hyperaemia.
- More likely to be seen in those children with delayed diagnosis or more aggressive subtypes especially if there is associated reduced mobility.
- In mild cases osteopenia can be a subjective phenomenon, but in more severe cases loss of bone density and thinning or 'pencilling' of the cortex can be marked.

Diffuse osteopenia
- Secondary to uncontrolled JIA, systemic corticosteroid therapy and immobilization of joint and limbs secondary to pain or a combination.
- Bone densitometry should be used in all children with suspected osteopenia.

Periostitis
- A periosteal reaction, classically in the digits, in the periosteum adjacent to the joint and extending along the diaphysis, most frequently seen in HLA-B27-associated disease.

Epiphyseal overgrowth
- Secondary to hypervascularity of the affected joint. The resultant overgrowth can lead to limb length discrepancy and secondary mechanical difficulties. At the knee this typically results in medial overgrowth of the distal tibia. Radiologically there may also be features of advanced bone age

Erosions and subchondral cysts
- Much rarer in JIA than in adult rheumatoid disease
- Absence of erosions does not exclude JIA

Ankylosis
- With modern treatment ankylosis should be rarely seen. In our experience plain radiographs in advanced uncontrolled disease will demonstrate joint space narrowing due to erosion of cartilage (Fig. 9.18).

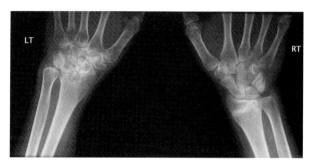

Fig. 9.18 Comparison image of two wrists. The left wrist demonstrates the marked loss of joint space and bony destruction of late JIA.

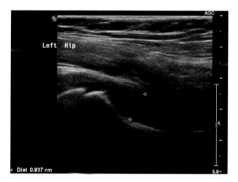

Fig. 9.19 Ultrasound of a 9mm hip effusion in a child with a flare of JIA symptoms. Note there is nothing to distinguish this effusion from septic arthritis or a reactive arthritis.

Ultrasound (US)
- Readily available and no radiation exposure (Fig. 9.19).
- Particularly useful for examining large joints, such as the hip, knee, and shoulder—will demonstrate effusions and synovial thickening.
- May be used to guide injection of certain joints, and can be used to diagnose ruptured popliteal cyst in the child presenting with calf swelling.

Magnetic resonance imaging (MRI)
- Excellent for demonstrating synovial disease (Figs 9.22, 9.23)
- Younger children will require sedation or general anaesthetic

Synovium
- In a normal joint, synovium is low/intermediate signal on T1W-weighted (T1W) and T2-nweighted (T2W) sequences.
- In the inflamed joint, the synovium thickens, and on T2W sequences becomes high signal and of similar signal to joint fluid.
- On non-contrast-enhanced T1W sequences synovium remains intermediate signal but enhances post-gadolinium contrast. Fat-suppressed T1W allows synovium to be seen clearly as high signal tissue.

Joint effusions
- Low signal on T1W and high signal on T2W and proton density sequences (Fig. 9.20).

Joint and articular cartilage
- Articular cartilage abnormalities are seen far earlier on MRI than plain films (Fig. 9.20).
- Cartilage abnormalities are not common in children with JIA, and occur in the knee of only around 10% of children with early disease. Visible erosions on MRI would further highlight the need for aggressive medical therapy to control synovitis (Fig. 9.21). Articular cartilage abnormalities consist of irregularity in the cartilage surfaces, fissures extending from the joint surface down to the subchondral bone, and generalized thinning. Focal abnormalities in the cartilage on T2W images are seen as high signal areas and fissures within the cartilage are seen as linear areas of high signal extending through the cartilage. Subchondral enhancement can also be identified which may represent increased vascularity, leading to overall cartilage thinning. Early changes in articular cartilage can be identified before erosions become obvious on standard sequences.

Meniscal hypoplasia
- Associated with larger effusions and a greater synovial thickness and volume.
- Loss of the normal triangular shape of the meniscus or 'hypoplasia' is an early sign that the meniscus is affected by disease.
- More chronically MRI can demonstrate more atrophic appearances or even complete absence of the menisci.

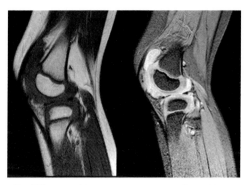

Fig. 9.20 Two MRI images of the knee of a child with JIA. On the T1-weighted image (left) the fluid and synovial thickening are intermediate signal. On the T2-weighted image (right) the joint fluid and synovium are high signal and can just be distinguished from the epiphyseal cartilage.

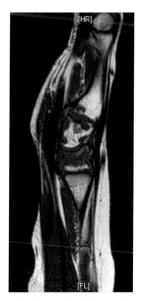

Fig. 9.21 A sagittal T1-weighted image of a child's wrist showing multiple erosions in the capitate. The marrow is white and the erosions are seen as irregular round subcortical lesions.

Bone marrow oedema
- Non-specific sign and is best identified on short TI inversion recovery (STIR)
- Bone marrow oedema is probably due to an increased vascularity in the marrow, leading to accumulation of fluid (Fig. 9.17).

Bony erosions
- Low signal areas on T1W sequences and are preceded by marrow oedema on fat-suppressed T2W images (Fig. 9.21).
- Once erosion has occurred, this is seen as high signal area on T2W images in the subchondral bone that demonstrates enhancement on T1W-weighted gadolinium images.

Computed tomography (CT)
Limited role in JIA. CT is sensitive at demonstrating alternative spinal pathology such as spondylolisthesis and spondylolysis.

May have a role in image guidance in injecting certain joints, e.g. temporomandibular and sacroiliac joints.

Other imaging modalities
Nuclear medicine
Limited role in JIA. Inflammation of a joint can be demonstrated during the blood pool phase with an increased distribution of tracer around an affected joint but this is non-specific.

Further reading
Petty RE, Southwood TR, Manners P *et al*. International League of Associations for Rheumatology classification of juvenile idiopathic arthritis: second revision, Edmonton, 2001. *J Rheumatol*. 2004; **31**:390–2.

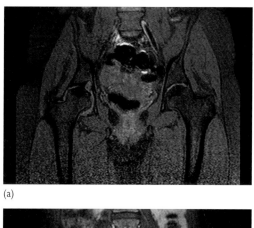

(a)

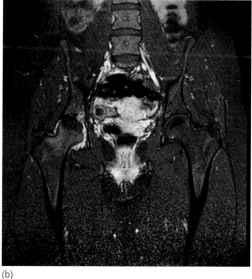

(b)

Fig. 9.22 (a) and (b) Coronal fat-suppressed T1-weighted images pre- and post-contrast. An older child with JIA and an acutely inflamed right hip. The thickened inflamed synovium around the right femoral head is relatively high signal on the pre-contrast images (as is often seen) but enhances vividly on the post-contrast images. This allows distinction from joint fluid which should be low signal on pre- and post-contrast T1-weighted images.

Imaging in inflammatory arthritis

Types of arthritis and imaging

Arthritis

The most important type of peripheral arthritis, in terms of frequency and impact, is rheumatoid arthritis. Other disorders include the various seronegative arthropathies (psoriatic arthritis, ankylosing spondylitis, and reactive arthritis), crystal arthritis (gout and pyrophosphate crystal deposition disease), arthritis in systemic connective tissue diseases, arthritis caused by infections and several uncommon disorders like pigmented villonodular synovitis. Most have readily identifiable features on imaging; some findings are diagnostic, some are prognostic and some are both.

Imaging modalities

Most musculoskeletal imaging focuses on plain X-rays. However, a number of techniques are available and the use of more complex procedures is increasing. The most recent change is the greater use of ultrasound, which is becoming an essential imaging approach in routine care.

The use of magnetic resonance imaging (MRI) in arthritis imaging is limited by its cost and relatively long examination times. Its clinical use is generally confined to certain types of arthritis such as septic arthritis, where it is important to delineate the extent of bone and soft-tissue involvement, or to certain joints which are poorly accessible to ultrasound such as sacroiliac joints.

Computed tomography (CT), isotope scans and dual energy X-ray absorptiometry (DEXA) are little used for arthritis.

Commonly used modalities

- Plain X-rays: standard method
- Ultrasound: increasingly used in routine care
- Magnetic resonance imaging (MRI): mainly research method

Little used modalities

- CT: limited value in peripheral joints
- Isotope scans: being replaced by ultrasound
- DEXA scans: limited value in peripheral joints

Use of imaging

Imaging has several aims in patients with arthritis. These comprise:

- Making the diagnosis
- Assessing severity and prognosis
- Defining response to treatment
- Surgical intervention
- Complications

Rheumatoid arthritis

Clinical features

Rheumatoid arthritis is a chronic inflammatory polyarthritis. It results in continuing symptoms from joint inflammation, structural joint damage, and consequent disability. Treatment aims to reduce synovial inflammation and to reduce the progression of joint damage and limit disability. Early diagnosis and subsequent early treatment are both important to limit the consequences of untreated synovial inflammation.

The characteristic features of rheumatoid arthritis relevant for imaging assessments involve:

- involvement of hands and feet
- symmetrical distribution
- persistence of joint inflammation
- erosive changes
- involvement of tendons and soft tissues
- progression towards joint destruction

Imaging modalities

Radiography

Erosions are the key finding for diagnosing rheumatoid arthritis. Erosions—defects in the surface of bones—often begin at the bare area of the joint not covered by cartilage. These marginal erosions reflect mechanical action of the hypertrophied synovium and pannus (granulation tissue). They are not diagnostic of rheumatoid arthritis as they occur in other conditions, but are typical. In the early stages of rheumatoid arthritis erosions are often ill defined.

Changes in rheumatoid arthritis on plain X-rays

- Soft-tissue swelling
- Periarticular osteopenia
- Loss of joint space
- Erosions
- Loss of alignment
- Joint destruction
- Secondary osteoarthritis

The distribution of changes is characteristic of rheumatoid arthritis. Usually they are symmetrical and involve the small joints of the hands and feet, particularly the metacarpophalangeal and metatarsophalangeal joints.

The progression of change is also typical of the disease. In the early phases there may be no more that soft-tissue swelling and osteopenia with a few scattered erosions. With time the extent and severity of erosive disease increases so that eventually there may be widespread joint destruction and ankylosis. Disease-modifying drugs and biological treatments reduce the progression of damage.

Simple scoring systems are available to assess progression. Though widely used in clinical trials they have not been adopted in routine practice. The commonest scoring systems are Sharp scores and Larsen scores, which have ranges of over 400 or 200. These scoring systems mainly focus on erosions.

Ultrasound (US)

High-resolution ultrasound is better than clinical examination and conventionnal X-rays in diagnosing and assessing joint and bursal effusion and synovitis. It is the imaging modality of choice for tendon pathology. It is also more sensitive in detecting erosions. The main changes seen on ultrasound comprise:

- Effusions
- Synovial swelling (synovitis)
- Tendonopathy
- Tendon rupture
- Erosions

In addition Doppler ultrasound, particularly power Doppler imaging, allows an assessment of synovial vascularity. It can therefore help distinguish inflamed and non-vascular synovial swelling.

Ultrasound imaging is most useful in the early stages of arthritis. Many clinicians use it to confirm the presence of synovial inflammation in patients in whom there is diagnostic uncertainty. It also helps define the extent of early disease and its severity and progression. In established arthritis it helps evaluate the extent of specific problems; for example the activity of synovitis in the feet or the severity of tendon disease in the hands.

Magnetic resonance imaging (MRI)

MRI provides excellent images in rheumatoid arthritis and can show soft-tissue changes, cartilage changes, bony erosions, and inflammatory change in the synovium. Gadolinium-based intravenous contrast agents are particularly useful in defining the extent and severity of synovial inflammation, though there are concerns about the risk of renal complications (nephrogenic systemic fibrosis when given to patients with pre-existing renal impairment). MRI is the most sensitive approach for identifying diagnostic and prognostic changes in early rheumatoid arthritis and for defining the benefits of early intensive treatment.

Other imaging modalities

Isotope scans highlight areas of active inflammation, particularly synovitis. In some patients they help identify synovitis when the diagnosis of rheumatoid arthritis is uncertain. With the advent of ultrasound they are rarely used.

CT and DEXA scans both show changes, and osteoporosis is commonplace in the disease, but they have limited diagnostic value.

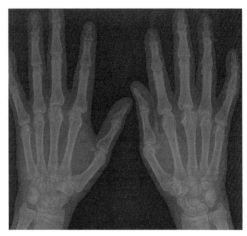

Fig. 10.1 Early severe rheumatoid arthritis.

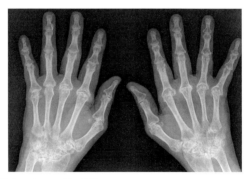

Fig. 10.2 Late rheumatoid arthritis.

Psoriatic arthritis

Clinical features

Psoriatic arthritis has similarities to rheumatoid arthritis, though usually less severe. Specific findings include inflammation at entheses—insertion of tendons or ligaments into bone—and dactylitis, colloquially termed 'sausage' fingers.

There are several subtypes of psoriatic arthritis:

- Distal interphalangeal joint only
- Asymmetric oligoarthritis (involving one or two joints)
- Polyarthritis: symmetric (similar to rheumatoid arthritis) or asymmetric
- Arthritis mutilans with deforming and destructive changes (very rare)
- Sacroiliac and spinal involvement (psoriatic spondylitis)

Imaging modalities

Radiography

The features are similar to rheumatoid arthritis but there is usually an asymmetric distribution, fewer joints are involved, progression is less marked and bone proliferation is common. The key changes comprise:

- Soft-tissue swelling
- Preserved periarticular bone density
- Joint space narrowing
- Bone erosion with marginal bony proliferation
- Bony proliferation including periarticular and shaft periostitis
- Osteolysis including 'pencil in cup' deformity and acroosteolysis (loss of terminal tufts of digits)
- Spur formation
- Malalignment, subluxation and ankylosis

The radiological findings reflect the clinical subtypes of psoriatic arthritis.

Ultrasound (US)

Ultrasound shows similar findings in psoriatic arthritis and rheumatoid arthritis. In addition, in psoriatic arthritis, it can show specific features such as enthesitis at the Achilles' tendon and comparable sites. It is also useful to assess dactylitis.

Magnetic resonance imaging (MRI)

This approach can show a variety of structural changes, especially when used in conjunction with contrast agents. These changes include:

- Bone erosion
- Bone oedema
- Synovitis
- Tendinopathy
- Extracapsular features of inflammation (including enthesitis)

Differences from rheumatoid arthritis

- Erosive changes irregular due to new bone formation
- Erosions progress to 'pencil in cup deformity' with marked osteolysis
- Asymmetrical erosions in the wrists and metacarpophalangeal joints
- Erosions of distal interphalangeal joints
- Periosteal and endosteal bone formation creates 'ivory' phalanx

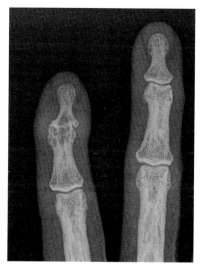

Fig. 10.3 Psoriatic arthritis affecting a distal interphalangeal joints.

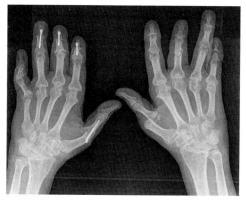

Fig. 10.4 Psoriatic arthritis showing 'arthritis mutilans' pattern after surgery.

Ankylosing spondylitis and reactive arthritis

Clinical features

The peripheral arthritis in these conditions is very similar. They overlap with psoriatic arthritis.

Ankylosing spondylitis mainly involves the spine and sacroiliac joints, but 20–30% of patients have peripheral arthritis. The knees, hips, and shoulders are usually involved.

Reactive arthritis, which follows an infective illness, is usually transient involving one or two large joints. However, the clinical pattern is variable. Occassional patients have a diffuse asymmetric arthritis and in some cases the hands and feet can be involved.

Both conditions can result in an enthesitis. Common sites include the Achilles tendon insertion, the insertion of the plantar fascia into the calcaneus, the tibial tuberosity, and the iliac crest. Dactylitis (sausage digits) occasionally occurs in reactive arthritis.

Imaging modalities

Radiography

In early disease X-rays are usually normal. Both loss of joint space and bone erosion are seen in the peripheral joints, though periarticular bone density is usually preserved. Proliferation around sites of erosion is more characteristic of ankylosing spondylitis.

In advanced disease periosteal reaction and proliferation at sites of tendon insertion are commonplace. One example is exuberant plantar spurs.

Magnetic resonance imaging (MRI)

Imaging of peripheral joints can show erosions and enthesitis that are not seen on plain X-rays. Imaging using gadolinium enhancement can show inflammatory lesions of enthesitis.

Ultrasound (US)

In active arthritis ultrasound shows similar changes of synovial inflammation to rheumatoid arthritis

In addition it can show sites of inflammation at the entheses, particularly in the foot and lower limb, such as the Achilles tendon. In these sites ultrasound can detect the two principal features of soft-tissue inflammation—tendon thickening and bursitis as well as hypervascularity using colour/power Doppler methods.

Gout

Clinical features

This common form of arthritis spans occasional acute episodes of monoar-thritis to a chronic inflammatory polyarthritis. It is due to uric acid accu-mulation. Its characteristic feature is gouty tophi—deposits of uric acid crystals—in many sites in the body.

Imaging modalities

Radiography

Subcutaneous tophi appear as asymmetric and lobulated soft-tissue masses. Intraosseous tophi frequently lead to bone erosions, which are well-defined with overhanging edges and without associated osteopenia. Compared with RA, joint space narrowing occurs late in disease. Ankylosis or joint space widening may also occur in advanced disease. Extraarticular erosions and osteolytic lesions have also been described.

Key features of gout, related to its duration, comprise:
- Early: asymmetric soft-tissue swelling around affected joint
- Intermediate: 'punched out' juxta-articular erosions
- Late: interosseous tophi, joint-space narrowing, deformities and sub-luxation with calcium deposits in the soft tissues

Ultrasound (US)

There is growing interest in the use of ultrasound to diagnose and assess gout. Recent findings indicate it can detect:
- Deposition of uric acid crystals on cartilaginous surfaces
- Periarticular tophaceous material
- Typical gouty erosions

Magnetic resonance imaging (MRI)

Imaging can detect all the key changes of gout and can be used to assess highly specific changes, such as decreases in the size of gouty tophi with treatment.

Pyrophosphate crystal deposition disease

Clinical features

Pyrophosphate crystal deposition disease is due to deposits of calcium phosphate crystals in joints. It has three main forms:
- acute synovitis, often termed pseudogout, often with chondrocalcinosis—finely stippled calcification in articular hyaline and fibrocartilage
- chronic arthritis, mimics rheumatoid arthritis or osteoarthritis, and commonly involves knees and wrists.
- asymptomatic findings of cartilage calcification

Imaging modalities

Radiography

Pyrophosphate crystal deposition disease results in number of characteristic features on plain X-rays. The presence of chondrocalcinosis is most characteristic, but other non-specific changes are equally important.

Characteristic radiographic features include:
- soft-tissue calcification
- joint space narrowing
- articular surface sclerosis
- subchondral cyst formation without osteophyte formation or bone growth
- large intraosseous geodes in occasional patients

Chondrocalcinosis is found in both fibrocartilage and hyaline articular cartilage. Common sites comprise of:
- menisci of the knee
- triangular cartilage of the wrist
- symphysis pubis

The distribution of radiographic involvement can help differentiate calcium pyrophosphate deposition disease from osteoarthritis. It affects joints not commonly involved in osteoarthritis. In the knee, tricompartmental involvement or isolated patellofemoral abnormalities are seen more commonly than with osteoarthritis. Cortical erosions on the femur superior to the patella and osteonecrosis of the medial femoral condyle may also be diagnostic clues.

Ultrasound (US)

This shows typical changes of inflammatory arthritis together with evidence of calcium pyrophosphate deposits. These give hyperechoic signals including:
- thin bands parallel to the surface of the hyaline cartilage
- 'punctate' pattern of thin spots in fibrous cartilage and tendons
- homogeneous nodular deposits in bursae and articular recesses

Magnetic resonance imaging (MRI)

Joint inflammation, damage and calcium pyrophosphate deposition can be imaged using MRI. It shows more involved articular surfaces and meniscal bodies than plain X-rays. Chondrocalcinosis in the articular cartilage is seen as linear and punctate hypointense regions.

Less common forms of arthritis

Systemic lupus erythematosus (□ p. 396)

Although lupus is a multisystem disorder, joint disease is frequent. In most patients it involves low-grade arthralgia needing only minimal therapy. In some patients (less than 5%) there is a deforming arthritis with erosions.

Some patients have marked ligamentous laxity, which can result in significant deformities in the hands and feet joints. These changes are often termed 'Jaccoud's arthritis'; they resemble the arthritis that follows rheumatic fever.

In some patients it is difficult to differentiate lupus from rheumatoid arthritis; these patients have erosive disease and are sometimes considered to have 'Rupus'.

The range of imaging changes in lupus includes:
• Juxta-articular osteopenia is common
• Scant and asymmetric joint erosions are well described
• Non-erosive carpal collapse is some patients
• Para-metacarpophalangeal hook formation in occasional cases

Other autoimmune rheumatic diseases

Scleroderma and overlap autoimmune rheumatic disorders often involve arthritis. When joint symptoms are present they are accompanied by a range of radiological changes which include:
• Periarticular osteoporosis
• Joint space narrowing
• Erosion
• Acro-osteolysis
• Flexion contracture
• Calcinosis

Septic arthritis

Infection should always be considered in patients with an acute monoarticular arthritis. Infection can arrive by hematogenous spread, direct inoculation or from operation.

Imaging modalities

Radiography

Initially plain X-rays show soft-tissue swelling and joint effusion. There may be joint space widening initially due to a tense effusion. Subsequently, as cartilage and bone is destroyed, joint space narrowing and marginal erosions are seen. Extensive joint destruction is seen in advanced cases.

Magnetic resonance imaging (MRI)

MRI is the most important imaging modality, especially when used with gadlinium enhancement. It shows joint effusion, destruction of cartilage, synovial thickening, cellulitis in surrounding soft tissues, and reactive marrow oedema. Synovial enhancement, perisynovial edema, and joint effusion can all be related to joint sepsis.

Other imaging modalities

Isotope scans are also useful to evaluate septic arthritis, particularly in the setting of joint replacement. 111-Indium-labelled white cell scans are particularly useful in this clinical situation.

Tuberculous arthritis

Tuberculous arthritis can involve any joint, but it has a predilection for large joints like the hip and knee. It usually involves one joint, but multiple lesions can occur. In most cases both synovium and periarticular bone are involved.

X-rays show soft-tissue swelling with loss of joint surface definition. With disease progression, marginal erosions may be seen. Periarticular bone loss may be striking. Cartilage loss and joint space destruction are late findings. Later in the disease, periosteal new bone formation may develop. The end stage is characterized by severe joint destruction and eventually sclerosis and fibrous ankylosis.

Magnetic resonance imaging shows are variety of changes:

- Focal cartilaginous destruction interspersed with relatively normal areas
- Chondral and subchondral bone erosions
- Bone marrow changes reflecting osteomyelitis or bone marrow oedema.
- Hypertrophied synovial lining
- Joint effusion
- Soft-tissue abnormalities (e.g. para-articular collections, myositis, tenosynovitis, bursitis, and sinus tract formation)

Pigmented villonodular synovitis

Pigmented villonodular synovitis is a locally aggressive proliferation of synovial joints, tendon sheaths and bursae. It often involves isolated, discrete lesions in tendon sheaths (particularly in the hand) and localized lesions in single joints, particularly the knee. In some patients there is diffuse involvement of the whole synovium of a large joint like the knee.

Imaging modalities

Radiography

Plain radiographs are normal in early disease. Subsequently they show a sof-tissue mass or joint effusion followed by erosions with a sclerotic rim and subchondral lucencies in advanced disease.

Magnetic resonance imaging (MRI)

Magnetic resonance imaging is the investigation of choice. It shows multiple synovial lesions of low signal intensity on all imaging sequences, and gradient echo images show apparently enlarged low signal masses (known as 'blooming artefact'). These features are due to the magnetic susceptibility properties of deposited haemosiderin.

Hydroxyapatite crystal disease

This is a disorder characterized by recurrent painful periarticular calcium hydroxyapatite deposits in tendons and soft tissues. It sometimes causes inflammatory arthritis.

Radiological changes include marked destructive changes and deformity in the affected joints, loss of joint space and attrition of subchondral bone. Areas of articular or periarticular calcification are often seen. Hydroxyapatite deposition should be considered when there is a destructive arthritis of the shoulder.

Remitting seronegative symmetrical synovitis with pitting oedema (RS3PE) syndrome

This distinct form of seronegative polyarthritis is characterized by late onset, symmetrical joint involvement, pitting oedema of hands and feet and good response to low-dose corticosteroids.

Imaging modalities

Plain X-rays are usually unremarkable. Ultrasound and magnetic resonance imaging both show evidence of symmetric subcutaneous oedema and synovitis of tendons and finger joints.

Hypertrophic osteoarthropathy

This comprises proliferative periostosis of the long bones, clubbing of fingers and synovitis. It is often seen in association with malignancies such as lung cancer or lymphoma.

Imaging modalities

Radiography

The key radiological finding is periosteal proliferation, which is single or laminated and often involves the tibia, fibula, radius, and ulna. Some patients have features of an inflammatory arthritis with soft-tissue swelling, joint effusion, and juxta-articular osteoporosis. Erosive changes are not seen.

Imaging in the autoimmune rheumatic diseases

Idiopathic inflammatory myopathies

Introduction
Idiopathic inflammatory myopathies (IIM) are rare acquired autoimmune disorders of muscle causing weakness, disability and potentially multi-system involvement (incidence 2 to 10 per million). The three main groups distinguishable clinically and histologically are polymyositis (PM), dermatomyositis (DM) both typically presenting with symmetrical proximal girdle weakness and inclusion body myositis (IBM).

Role of imaging
Imaging is not included in the Peter and Bohan diagnostic criteria for IIM (1975) which is non-validated but MRI maybe indicated in the following circumstances:
• Diagnostic uncertainty e.g. normal CK (creatine kinase) /EMG (electro-myelogram) /suspected pyomyositis
• Determine optimal site for muscle biopsy
• Assess extent of inflammatory activity rather than irreversible damage.

Imaging modalities
Magnetic resonance imaging (MRI)
The imaging technique of choice.
• Sensitivity up to 100%
• Specificity 88%
• Positive predictive value 77%
• Negative predictive value 100%
• Active inflammation best seen on T2-weighted fat-suppressed short time inversion recovery (STIR) sequence as high signal, may appear normal on T1 image.
• Gadolinium may show inflammatory vascularization.
• Chronic atrophy/fibrotic scarring best seen on T1 image.
• Non-invasive, may avoid potentially painful EMG.
• Maybe abnormal in cases of amyopathic dermatomyositis.
• Higher muscle biopsy yield when biopsy site indicated by active lesion.
• There maybe limited availability in some hospitals.

Current research tools
Magnetic resonance spectroscopy (MRS)
This non-invasive method records the amount of specific chemical entities by their resonance in a defined volume of tissue.
  Phosphorus-31 (P31-MRS) monitors the oxidative metabolism of muscle by quantifying adenosine triphosphate (ATP), phosphocreatine (PCr) and inorganic phosphates (Pi).
• In myositis levels of PCr and ATP are lower on average than in controls at rest and following exercise.
• Levels correlate with clinically observed weakness and disability but not with MRI.
• Levels abnormal in patients with amyopathic dermatomyositis indicating inefficient metabolism during intense exercise.

Using proton MRS an abnormally low lipid-to-water ratio at onset of myositis due to oedema is seen, this is abnormally high after 3 months of treatment compared to controls and the clinical usefulness of this is unclear.

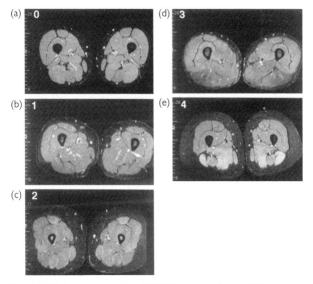

Fig. 11.1 MRI changes in myositis on MRI STIR sequence. (a) normal, (b) severe and homogenously abnormal signal intensity of the biceps femoris, semimembranosus, adductor magnus.

Reproduced from Lafforgue P, Janand Delenne B, Lassman-Vague V, Daumen-Legre V, Pham T, Vague P (1999). Painful swelling of the thigh in a diabetic patient: diabetic muscle infarction. *Diabet. Metab.* **25**, 255–60, with permission from Elsevier.

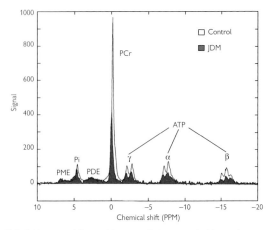

Fig. 11.2 P-31spectra of the quadriceps muscle in a control subject and a severely weakened patient with juvenile DM at rest. Peaks for the inorganic phosphate (Pi), phosphomonoesters (PME), phosphodiesters (PDE), phosphocreatine (PCr) and the αβ peaks of ATP are shown.

Reproduced from Park JH, Niermann KJ, Ryder NM, Nelson AE, Das A, Lawton AR, Hernanz-Schulman M, Olsen NJ (2000). Muscle abnormalities in juvenile dermatomyositis patients: P-31 magnetic resonance spectroscopy studies. *Arthritis Rheum.* **43**, 2359–2367. Reprinted with permission of John Wiley & Sons, Inc.

Systemic sclerosis

Introduction

Systemic sclerosis (SSc) is a rare condition with a pathological triad of immune disorder, vascular pathology, and fibrosis resulting in heterogenous clinical manifestations.

Skin fibrosis (e.g. sclerodactyly) is the hallmark feature, the extent of skin involvement allows classification into diffuse (30%) and limited subsets which help stratify risk of major organ-based complications, e.g. interstitial lung disease, renal crisis, pulmonary hypertension, gastrointestinal and cardiac involvement.

Role of imaging

A variety of imaging techniques are used to assess the pattern of organ involvement in SSc which indicates prognosis, directs management and contributes to SSc having the highest case-specific mortality of the auto-immune disorders.

Table 11.1 Organ-based investigation of systemic sclerosis

Respiratory	CXR, PFTs[*], HRCT, BAL
Cardiac	CXR, ECG[*], Echo Doppler[*], PFT[*]
Right heart Catheter	
Renal	US, Isotope GFR, Biopsy
Gastrointestinal	BA Swallow, Oesophageal scintigraphy
Endoscopy (upper/lower)	
Manometry (oesophageal, anal) Ba Follow through, Endo-anal ultrasound	

[*]Screening maybe advocated e.g. 6 monthly for the first 3 years since onset of diffuse SSc then annually and annually for limited SSc subset.

CXR, chest X-ray; BAL, bronchoalveolar lavage; PFT, pulmonary function tests; HRCT, high resolution computed tomography.

Imaging modalities

Radiography
- Soft-tissue calcinosis
- Acro-osteolysis

Calcinosis typically occurs at pressure areas, e.g. fingertips, may be complicated by ulceration and can be extensive. Acro-osteolysis of the distal phalanges maybe due to chronic underperfusion causing bone resorption.

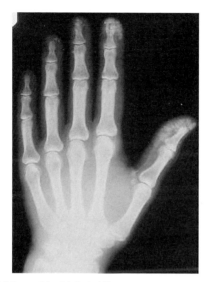

Fig. 11.3 Soft tissue calcinosis in limited SSc.

Reproduced from Isenberg D and Renton P (eds) (2003). *Imaging in Rheumatology. Oxford*: Oxford University Press.

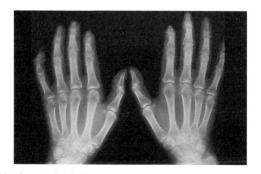

Fig. 11.4 Acroosteolysis in SSc.

Reproduced from Isenberg D and Renton P (eds) (2003). *Imaging in Rheumatology. Oxford*: Oxford University Press.

Peripheral vascular system imaging

Cutaneous blood flow measurement
- Laser Doppler flowmetry
- Infra-red thermographic assessment of cold induced spasm.

Angiography
- Corkscrew collaterals in vasa vasorum in Buerger's
- Distal tapering arteries in Buerger's
- No collaterals typically seen in SSc.
- Raynaud's phenomenon is almost universal in SSc due to vasospasm and underlying small vessel attenuation.

If atypical features are present, e.g. unilateral or fixed ischaemia (without preceding episodic pattern) or marked lower limb involvement other causes of vascular insufficiency should be excluded, e.g. large vessel thromboembolic disease, vasculitis, thromboangiitis obliteran (Buerger's disease). See Fig. 11.5.

Gastrointestinal imaging

The entire gut can be affected by fibrosis and dysmotility. Symptoms range from reflux and dysphagia of solids, postprandial fullness to delayed gastric emptying, abdominal bloating and diarrhoea due to small bowel bacterial overgrowth, constipation, pseudo-obstruction, and anal incontinence (see Table 11.2).

Renal imaging

The scleroderma renal crisis (SRC) is one of the most serious complications of SSc occurring in up to 10% of patients with the diffuse subset, often within the first 3 years, associated with death and reduced kidney survival. Patients may present with abrupt onset accelerated hypertension and acute renal failure, which may be associated with microangiopathic haemolytic anaemia (MAHA) on blood film.

Clinical diagnosis of SRC should be confirmed by renal biopsy once the blood pressure is at a safe level.

Ultrasound (renal)
- May exclude intercurrent renal disease.
- May determine site for biopsy.

Intravenous contrast studies should not be performed due to potential nephrotoxicity.

Nuclear medicine studies maybe used to gauge renal function accurately by ethylenediaminetetraacetic acid (EDTA) clearance.

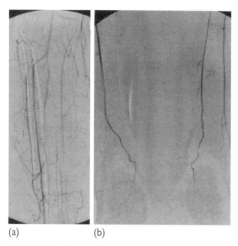

(a)   (b)

Fig. 11.5 (a) and (b) digital subtraction angiography in Buerger's disease/systematic sclerosis(SSc).

Reproduced from Isenberg D and Renton P (eds) (2003). *Imaging in Rheumatology*. Oxford: Oxford University Press.

Table 11.2 Imaging of gastrointestinal disease in SSc

Barium swallow	Reduced lower oesophageal sphincter tone, featureless wall, strictures, usually benign
Oesophagogastroscopy or if dilatation is required	Perform if mucosal/malignant lesion suspected
Oesophageal manometry	
Oesophogeal scintigraphy not commonly used	
Barium follow-through	Mid-gut lumen dilatation, featureless bowel wall, slowing of barium passage
Stacked coin appearance—prominent jejunal diverticulae due to muscle atrophy and dilatation	
Barium enema	Should avoid may cause prolonged contrast retention and severe constipation
Colonoscopy	Perform if rectal bleeding/unexpected weight loss Beware some increased risk of perforation
Anorectal ultrasound	Sphincter deficiencies associate with incontinence, more practical than MRI of pelvic floor

Respiratory imaging

Respiratory complications such as interstitial lung disease account for the majority of SSc-associated deaths so early diagnosis is essential; increased risks of pulmonary infection and carcinoma also contribute to mortality.

Chest radiograph
- Often normal or non-specific changes.
- Main value in excluding other pathology.

High resolution computed tomography (HRCT)
Uses 1mm scanning windows at 10mm intervals, evaluating 10% of lung tissue, rather than 1cm contiguous scans.

Investigation of choice in showing interstitial lung disease, often performed at diagnosis of diffuse SSc or if new respiratory symptoms develop or screening PFTs have declined.
- Prone positioning avoids physiological pooling of oedema which may misleadingly appear like alveolitis.
- Potentially reversible inflammation typically has a ground-glass appearance which is basal, bilateral, peripheral and posterior.
- Established, irreversible fibrosis may have a reticular pattern with architectural distorsion, cyst formation, and traction bronchiectasis.
- A mixture of active inflammation and chronic damage may be seen.
- Limited serial scans of involved levels allows monitoring, reduces radiation exposure.
- Changes correlate well with histological classification and prognosis, lung biopsies are not usually required.
- SSc mostly associates with non-specific interstitial pneumonia (NSIP) pattern which is more responsive to steroids with a better prognosis than usual interstitial pneumonia (UIP).

Bronchalveolar lavage maybe helpful but is not routine (Fig. 11.6).

Pulmonary vascular imaging

Chest radiograph
May be normal early on, or show prominent pulmonary arteries and peripheral pruning of vascular markings, then hilar prominence, lung fields are clear in primary subtypes.

Transthoracic Doppler echocardiography
A useful non-invasive screening tool for detection of pulmonary hypertension which is still severely life-limiting despite licensed therapies; this, may be secondary to lung fibrosis or primary, e.g. in limited SSc, years after onset.

Indicated in a patient complaining of unexplained breathlessness and with an isolated fall in transfer factor of the lung for carbon monoxide (TLCO).

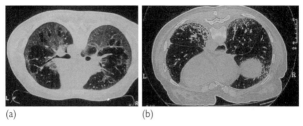

(a)   (b)

Fig. 11.6 (a) and (b) HRCT acute alveolitis/established fibrosis.
The decision on whether to treat interstitial lung disease is based upon the extent of disease on CT and TLCO, if less than 20% of the lung is abnormal on CT and TLCO more than 70%, careful observation and serial testing may be indicated.

Reproduced from Isenberg D and Renton P (eds) (2003). *Imaging in Rheumatology*. Oxford: Oxford University Press.

Right heart catheterization
Required to establish a diagnosis, performed at a designated pulmonary hypertension centre.

Cardiac imaging
Transthoracic echocardiography
- Pericardial disease uncommon, rarely associated with tamponade.
- Cardiac myositis uncommon, may occur in overlap syndromes.

Electrocardiogram may show dysrhythmia or conduction block.

Systemic lupus erythematosus

Introduction

Systemic lupus erythematosus (SLE) is an autoimmune rheumatic disease mostly affecting women of childbearing age which can affect virtually every organ in the body, most commonly the skin and joints.

The American College of Rheumatology produced classification criteria (revised 1997, see http://www.rheumatology.org) which do not include any imaging, these are not diagnostic criteria but do include the typical features of SLE.

Role of imaging

A wide variety of imaging methods maybe used to confirm clinically suspected organ complications of SLE to direct management.

Musculoskeletal imaging

Radiography

Arthralgia is common (90%), non-erosive arthritis may occur but X-ray abnormalities are uncommon and the presence or severity of these does not correlate with disease activity.

• Periarticular demineralization	40%	Subluxation	5–10%
• Soft tissue swelling	20%	Erosion	< 10%
• Avascular necrosis[*]	5–10%	Bone infarction[†]	rare

[*]E.g. femur, navicular, metacarpals, lumbar vertebrae
[†]May appear as dense, irregular shadows resembling puffs of smoke in the metaphysodiaphyseal regions of long bones.
Joint space narrowing, distal phalanx sclerosis, extra-articular calcification may occur.

Magnetic resonance imaging (MRI)

Avascular necrosis (AVN)

• MRI is the investigation of choice
• Risk factors include steroid use
• Features of hip AVN include:
  • Focal deficit in anterosuperior margin of femoral head, characteristically (80%) but not pathognomically bounded by a low signal margin, signalling the interface between viable and necrotic bone.
  • 'Double-line signal' is a high signal-intensity rim within the low-signal margin, representing hyperaemic zone and granulation tissue.

Osteomyelitis

• Sensitivity and specificity 90–100%
• Gadolinium-enhanced MRI may distinguish osteomyelitis (cortical defects, abnormal marrow and soft tissue) from acute medullary bone infarction(thin linear rim enhancement)

Bone scintigraphy

• Uncommonly used in SLE
• Sensitive for AVN/osteomyelitis but not as specific as MRI, uses radiation.
• In SLE arthropathy may be normal or mild increased uptake compared to marked increase in rheumatoid arthritis.

Dual energy absorptiometry (DEXA) scanning
- Standard lumbar spine/hip views used to assess bone mineral density.
- SLE carries a fivefold increased fracture risk compared to control population, damage restricting mobility and steroid use are risk factors.

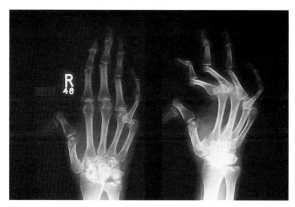

Fig. 11.7 Plain radiograph—Jaccoud's arthropathy. Shows ulnar deviation, MCP subluxation, but no erosions, differentiating this from the joint destruction of rheumatoid arthritis. The deformities can be associated with SLE, on examination they are correctable, related to supporting structures and possibly capsular inflammation.

Reproduced from Isenberg D and Renton P (eds) (2003). *Imaging in Rheumatology*. Oxford: Oxford University Press.

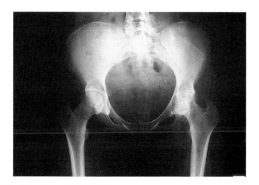

Fig. 11.8 Plain radiograph, AVN hip.

Reproduced from Isenberg D and Renton P (eds) (2003). *Imaging in Rheumatology*. Oxford: Oxford University Press.

Cardiovascular imaging

Pericardial disease is the most common cardiac abnormality seen in SLE which can also cause myocardial, endocardial or valvular involvement and accelerated atherogenesis.

Transthoracic echocardiography (echo)

Pericardial disease

- Pericardial thickening or effusion may be seen.
- Evident more commonly on echo (37%) than clinically (29%).
- Therapeutic pericardiocentesis possible if tamponade present.
- Pericardial thickening may appear weeks after an effusion due to constrictive pericarditis (rare), cardiac catheterization or thoracotomy maybe needed to make definitive diagnosis.

Myocardial disease

- Myocarditis occurs in up to 15% patients clinically but up to 80% of post-mortem studies.
- Global or regional hypokinesis may occur and can occur reversibly with generalized flares.
- Left ventricular diastolic function may cause abnormal prolongation of isovolumic relaxation (>100ms), which is an early marker correlating with active disease on Doppler studies.
- Technetium-99m Sestamibi (Tc-99m MIBI) and single photon emission computerised tomography (SPECT) might be more sensitive for myocardial perfusion defects (reported abnormal in up to 40% of asymptomatic patients).

Valvular disease

Systolic murmurs occur in up to a third of patients with SLE, diastolic less often. They maybe associated with fever, anaemia, hypertension in addition to valvulopathy which can be distinguished into three groups. The classical Libman and Sachs endocarditis (1924) occurs in up to 50% at post-mortem.

Valvular abnormalities may frequently appear, resolve, or persisting ones may change between repeated studies, those affected have greater morbidity and mortality but lesions do not associate with duration, activity or severity of SLE (see Table 11.3).

Coronary artery disease

SLE is associated with a generally increased risk of coronary artery disease and up to 50-fold in the 35–44yrs age group compared to age-matched control population for reasons that are not fully explained by conventional risk factors.

Ischaemic symptoms can occur due to coronary vasculitis ('simple' inflammation of the blood vessel wall), which has no definitive diagnostic features on angiography so myocardial perfusion tests maybe necessary to distinguish this from atherosclerosis (accumulation of lipids on the inner vessel wall leading to plaque formation and often subsequent rupture; inflammation is now known to be involved in the process). Although typical angiographic appearances of vasculitis include aneurysmal dilatation and elongated smooth lesions, it can be difficult to differentiate from atherogenesis, cardiac MRI and SPECT may be useful.

Table 11.3 Features of vegetations associated with SLE on transthoracic echocardiography

| | Valvular vegetations | | Diffuse valvular thickening* | Variable |
	Sterile	Infected		
Thickening	Distinct, irregular		Diffuse thickening ≥1 leaflet	Localized part/all leaflet
Shape	Scalloped 'brush-like'	Pedunculated	Dome shaped	
		2–4mm		Flattening diastolic slope
Attachment	Proximal/middle leaflet tip portion			
to valve	Mitral/aortic			
Movement	Do not move independently	Chaotic flapping		
Valve function	Do not affect	May affect	Stenosis/ regurgitation	May regurgitate

Transoesophageal doppler echocardiography (TOE) is superior to transthoracic echo in detecting vegetations e.g. showing incidence of 74% valvular abnormality, 50% diffuse thickening in SLE irrespective of antiphospholipid antibody status.

Regurgitation is more common than stenosis, with masses found on the atrial side of the mitral valve or on the vessel side of the aortic valve.

Thoracic imaging

Up to 50–70% patients have thoracic disease directly due to SLE which can involve the pleura, lung parenchyma, airways, pulmonary vasculature, and respiratory muscles or secondary to other disease complications e.g. effusion of nephrotic disease.

Pleural disease

Up to 60% patients have pleurisy clinically, up to 80% at post-mortem.

- Pleural effusion maybe present 16–50% on chest radiograph, generally small (21% seen on HRCT) can be bilateral in up to 50% cases.

Pulmonary disease

Up to 50% patients affected.

- Chest radiograph maybe normal
- HRCT usually needed to demonstrate parenchymal abnormalities, which may occur prior to symptom onset or decline in PFTs.
- Elevated hemidiaphragm may be due to respiratory muscle dysfunction (see Table 11.4)

Respiratory infection

Infection has to be excluded in any SLE patient presenting with new pulmonary symptoms with pulmonary infiltrates because SLE carries a threefold increased risk of infection, including common bacteria and opportunistic pathogens.

The chest radiograph may show multiple patchy abnormalities or cavitating nodules. Infections include pulmonary tuberculosis, increased rates of *Staphylococcus*, *Pneumocystis carinii* and potentially fatal nocardia.

Pulmonary haemorrhage

Rare but with mortality of at least 50%.

- Chest radiograph shows ill-defined patchy, acinar opacities typically bilateral in the lower zones, normailizing within a few days after bleeding stops.
- Early CT changes include uniform nodules of 1–3mm throughout zones, acute exacerbations can show ground glass changes.

Pulmonary vasculature

Pulmonary arterial hypertension (PAH) reported in 14% cases, can be secondary to interstitial fibrosis, less commonly due to recurrent pulmonary emboli associated with anti-phospholipid antibodies.

- Chest radiograph maybe normal early on but develops right ventricular and pulmonary arteries (hilar) enlargement with pruning of distal arteries.
- Echo may show raised right ventricle pressure

Ventilation/perfusion (V/Q) or CT pulmonary angiogram (CTPA) maybe needed to exclude a pulmonary embolus.

Table 11.4 Radiographic features of pulmonary disease associated with SLE

Acute pneumonitis / Non-infective	Chronic interstitial disease	Bronchiolitis obliterans	organizing pneumonia (BOOP)*	Non-specific interstitial pneumonia (NSIP)
1–4%	Clinically rare <3%		Rare, subacute	Subacute
Patchy consolidation†	radiographically 6%	Bilateral	Patchy consolidation	
Basal infiltrates	CXR may be normal	scattered ground glass	subpleural ground glass	
Focal atelectasis	bi-basal irregular linear opacities		air space consolidation irregular linear opacities	

Table 11.4 (Contd)

	ground-glass	(alveolitis)		all zones		bronchial dilatation
Elevated diaphragm	honeycombing (damage)		subpleural (50%)‡	lower zone		
Pleural effusion				subpleural thickening (damage)		
				septal thickening		
				mild mediastinal adenopathy		
				discrete nodules		

*In this small airways disease the parenchyma is spared not involved as in BOOP. The CXR maybe normal or show mild hyperinflation, or peripheral attenuation of vascular markings. The HRCT shows focal, well defined areas of decreased lung attenuation associated with vessels of decreased calibre, bronchiectasis or centrilobular opacities maybe seen.

†Indistinguishable radiographic appearance of patchy consolidation, atelectasis, possible concomitant effusion which could also be due to infection, pulmonary haemorrhage, pulmonary embolism.

‡Other features include bronchial dilatation within consolidation, discrete centrilobular nodules, mediastinal lymphadenopathy, pleural effusions. PFT's show restrictive deficit. Pulmonary haemorrhage is rare, varies from mild to life-threatening forms with mortality of at least 50%. CXR show ill-defined patchy, acinar-opacities typically bilateral and in lower zones, but unilateral/asymmetrical forms can occur. The CXR usually normalizes within a few days after bleeding stops. Early CT changes include uniform nodules of 1–3mm throughout zones, acute exacerbations can show ground-glass changes.

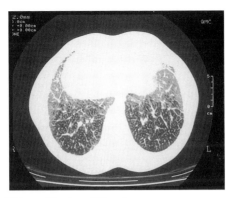

Fig 11.9 CT chest—diffuse interstitial lung disease.

Reproduced from Isenberg D and Renton P (eds) (2003). *Imaging in Rheumatology*. *Oxford*: Oxford University Press.

Neuromuscular imaging

Diaphragmatic elevation with progressive loss of lung volume 'shrinking lung syndrome' is a well-recognized though rare radiological abnormality in SLE, associated with dyspnoea and restrictive lung function tests.

Renal imaging

30–50% of patients with SLE will develop glomerulonephritis, this diagnosis requires a renal biopsy for confirmation and prognostic purposes.

Ultrasound (US)
- May be normal.
- Kidneys may appear small (<9cm) with increased echogenicity.
- Hypoechoic cortical rim representing cortical interstitial oedema or acute necrosis is rare.
- Doppler US picks up signals form intrarenal arcuate arteries in corticomedullary region allows measurement of resistance index (RI).
- RI may correlate with creatinine level, interstitial disease and chronicity index which is predictive of poor outcome.

Ethyldiaminetetraacetic acid (EDTA) clearance study
This measures renal function more accurately than can be calculated using the Cockcroft–Gault method.

Gastrointestinal imaging

Up to two-thirds of patients with SLE develop gastrointestinal symptoms during their illness, any part of the gut or hepatobiliary system can be affected.

It has been reported that 50% of patients experience abdominal pain throughout their lifetime, the majority due to common conditions, e.g. cholecystitis, but SLE specific problems include serositis, mesenteric ischaemia, pneumatoses intestinalis from necrotizing enterocolitis, and hepatobiliary abnormalities, rarely small vessel gut vasculitis of small/large bowel causing infarction, perforation or peritonitis occur.

A low threshold for investigation necessary because steroid use risks gut ulceration, impaired peritoneal defence mechanism, wound healing and increased risk of infection.

Inflammatory bowel disease is as common as in the background population, coeliac is a little more common and there is increased risk of infection, e.g. salmonella, invasive amoebic colitis, but no known increase in tumours (see Table 11.5).

Table 11.5 Radiographic imaging in the investigation of abdominal pain in SLE (adapted from Al-Hakeem and McMillen[1].)

Region of pain	Investigation
Mid-epigastric or shoulder	Plain radiograph or CT abdomen with contrast (for free air or leak)
Right upper quadrant	Plain radiograph (for free air) and US (image gallbladder) or CT abdomen with contrast (for free air or leak)
Left lower quadrant	CT abdomen with contrast (for free air or leak)
Right lower quadrant	US (of appendix) and/or CT abdomen with contrast
Diffuse abdominal	US and/or CT abdomen prior to starting steroids (if no signs of sepsis)

Other imaging modalities

Oesophagogastroduodenoscopy maybe useful for peptic ulcer disease.

Doppler US of superior mesenteric artery+/– portal vein maybe useful for bowel ischaemia but is observer-dependent and technically difficult.

Visceral angiography maybe useful in the diagnosis of bowel ischaemia but may not show small vessel vasculitis and may exacerbate renal dysfunction.

Gallium/white cell scan may highlight source of sepsis/inflammation if otherwise unidentified.

Laparotomy considered if:

Patient has diffuse abdominal pain and sepsis

Patient has focal peritonitis or history consistent with perforated ulcer, cholecystitis, or diverticulitis, but laparoscopy maybe preferable if SLE is very active

[1] Al-Hakeem, MS, and McMillen, MA (1998). Evaluation of abdominal pain in systemic lupus erythematosus. *Am J Surg*, **176**, 291–4.

Neurological imaging

Neuropsychiatric lupus (NPSLE) can affect up to 75% patients, has a wide clinical spectrum and is diagnostically challenging.

Imaging of the brain may help distinguish differential diagnoses and indicate prognosis, MRI is the anatomical investigation of choice.

Functional modalities may be more sensitive than anatomical which may show non-specific findings.

Computed tomography (CT)
- May be abnormal in 25–29% pts, cerebral atrophy most commonly.
- Inferior to MRI, only use when MRI not available or contraindicated.
- Most useful for showing large infarcts, intracerebral haemorrhage, massive brain oedema and excluding brain abscess, meningeal enhancement, mass lesions, mycotic lesions.
- Not sensitive for non-focal presentations, e.g. seizure, confusion, depression, altered cognition.
- Insensitive to chronic white-matter disease, small infarcts, transverse myelitis, punctuate lesions, diffuse brain injury and leucoencephalopathy.

Magnetic resonance imaging (MRI) (see Fig. 11.3)
- Sensitive to infarcts, haemorrhage, transverse myelitis.
- Up to 75% patients with active NPSLE will have abnormal MRI, but most lesions do not represent acute/active disease but old injury.
- Acute lesions on T2-weighted images suggesting active SLE include new infarction, discrete grey matter lesions, diffuse grey matter intensities and cerebral oedema.
- New lesions or resolution of lesions or their enhancement following gadolinium on repeat scanning suggest active disease.
- An MRI should be obtained within 24h of the acute neurological event because the typical, reversible, high-intensity lesions associated with diffuse presentations resolve rapidly with corticosteroid therapy.
- Chronic lesions found in 25–50% SLE patients especially with increasing disease severity, age, and history of NPSLE.
- Most common chronic lesions are small focal subcortical white matter lesions (especially frontoparietal) which may represent neuronal injury.
- Less often cortical atrophy, periventricular white matter changes, ventricular dilatation, diffuse white matter changes, infarcts are seen.
- Increased sensitivity may come from quantitative T2-weighted measurements of grey matter and cerebral blood flow or MRS.

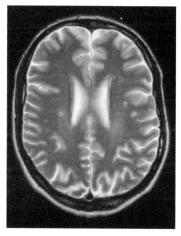

Fig 11.10 MRI brain—small vessel white-matter lesions—vasculitis.

Magnetic resonance spectroscopy (MRS)
- Research tool rather than mainstream clinical use partly due to limited availability.
- Proton MRS.
- This provides data in the form of absolute concentrations or a ratio of neuronal signalling molecules, e.g. N-acetylaspartic acid which maybe reduced in SLE and suggest injury.
- 31Phosphorus MRS.
- Assesses the pH, tissue energetics and phosphorus containing compounds in the brain, including those in membrane synthesis and breakdown.
- Decreased ATP and PCr in deep white matter seen in NPSLE, reversible with steroids and potentially consistent with ischaemia, neuronal death.

Positron emission tomography (PET)
- May not provide any further clinically useful information beyond that of MRI.
- Quantifies glucose uptake and use, using 1-(18F)-fluoro-2-deoxyglucose, other agents can assess oxygen uptake or cerebral blood flow.
- PET often abnormal in active NPSLE, e.g. with multiple focal defects in parietal–occipital with normal CT/MRI.
- Lesions may improve following steroid therapy, suggesting they represent hypometabolism, or ischaemia in active SLE but lesions seen in non-NPSLE patients too.

Angiography
- Available in a variety of formats, e.g. conventional, digital, subtracted, CT, or MR) but often normal in NPSLE, so rarely used.
- Magnetic resonance angiography (MRA) may be helpful to investigate medium-large vessel vasculitis.

Single-photon emission computed tomography (SPECT)
- Not recommended for routine clinical use but research.
- Sensitive e.g. 99Tc-HMPAO SPECT is abnormal in 86–100% patients with major NPSLE but poor specificity, 10–50% SLE patients without SLE.
- Most common abnormality in NPSLE is multiple small sites of decreased uptake suggested of patchy hypoperfusion.
- Hypoperfusion most often seen in territory of middle cerebral artery affecting parietal lobe (65–80%), frontal lobes (46–57%), basal ganglia (12–30%).
- Abnormalities can be more pronounced in more severely affected patients but poor differentiator of pathology, poor correlation with MRI.

Antiphospholipid syndrome

Introduction

The antiphospholipid syndrome (APS) was originally delineated in the 1980s and comprises vascular thrombosis and/or pregnancy morbidity in the presence of antiphospholipid antibodies (aPL) e.g. anticardiolipin (aCL) or anti-betaglycoprotein antibodies or lupus anticoagulant.

This maybe 'secondary' when associated with a systemic autoimmune disease most commonly SLE or 'primary' when in isolation. The internationally agreed Sapporo preliminary classification criteria for definite APS was published in 1999, revised in 2006 requiring laboratory and clinical fulfillment positive predictive value of 0.95.

Role of imaging

The accurate diagnosis of venous thromboembolism is essential because if APS is untreated there is a 20–70% risk of recurrent thrombosis whilst warfarinization carries a low risk of life-threatening bleeding.

APS may affect virtually any organ and thus a wide spectrum of imaging techniques are employed to manage patients.

Venous imaging

Table 11.6 Imaging used to diagnose deep venous thrombosis (DVT)

	Venogram	Ultrasound*	Impedance plethysmography‡	MRI
Sensitivity	100%	89–96% proximal DVT	71–98%	94.8% proximal DVT
	73%	below knee DVT		
Specificity	100%	86–100%	73–98%	95–100%
Advantages	Accuracy	Non-invasive	Non-invasive	Non-invasive
	Safe	Safe	Accurate	
	No contrast	May detect recurrent DVT	Identify alternative diagnosis	
	Widely available	90% return to normal at 1 yr		
		Positive predictive value 80% 2nd DVT		
Disadvantages	Invasive	Remain abnormal at 1yr in 50%	Not widely available	Expensive
	Contrast allergy	Difficult to detect recurrence	Operator dependent	Claustophobia
	7% minor side effects	Lower sensitivity calf DVT	Lower sensitivity calf DVT	Contraindications
	Caution in renal failure	Unreliable in low flow states	e.g. metallic implants	

*Ultrasound is the investigation of choice to visualize the deep veins failure of the veins to collapse with gentle pressure indicates the presence of clot.

†20–30% of these may extend thus repeat US 1–2 weeks maybe advocated. This strategy leads to 1–2% additional pick up of DVT and less than 1% symptomatic DVT/PE at 3 months in those with normal scans.

‡This non-invasive method was developed in 1969 based on the principle that the volume of blood in the leg affects electrical resistance. Electrodes placed across the calf, impedance is measured, this drops as a cuff is inflated around the thigh, on release of the cuff, there is a sudden rush of blood proximally and impedance rises rapidly but the presence of a clot the rise in impedance will be slower.

Respiratory imaging

Table 11.7 Imaging used to diagnose pulmonary embolism

	Pulmonary angiography (PA)	Ventilation/ perfusion scan* (V/Q)	Computed tomography/ pulmonary angiography (CTPA)
Sensitivity	100%	98%	94% for main/ segmental arteries, sensitivity 72% all sized arteries
Specificity	100%	10%	95%
Advantages	Accuracy	Less invasive	High negative predictive value
	Gold standard	Positive predictive value 88%	Make other diagnoses
Disadvantages	Invasive	High proportion non-diagnostic scan	May miss subsegmental thrombi[†]
	Contrast allergy/side effectsReported as probability	Contrast allergy/ side effects	
	63% interobserver variability Intermediate/Low 33%/13% PE on PA	Expense	

*V/Q scan first line investigation if CXR normal, if not CTPA.

[†]Clinical significance of subsegmental thrombi unclear, but may relate to recurrence and be relevant in APS. Multidetector CT may pick up these lesions.

Up to 60% V/Q scans non-diagnostic if CXR abnormal compared to 13% if CXR normal.

Contrast-enhanced Magnetic resonance angiography (MRA): data suggests this method has similar sensitivity and specificity to spiral CT but this requires further evaluation. The advantage is the use of gadolinium as a non-iodine contrast which is not nephrotoxic.

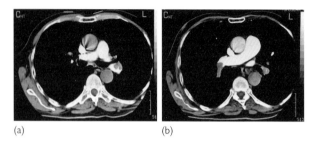

(a)   (b)

Fig. 11.11 Pulmonary embolism on spiral CT.
Reproduced from Isenberg D and Renton P (eds) (2003). *Imaging in Rheumatology*. Oxford: Oxford University Press.

Neurological imaging

The range of neuropsychiatric manifestations of APS varies from focal symptoms attributable to specific anatomical lesions to diffuse or global dysfunction.

Sneddon's syndrome is characterized by livedo reticularis and multiple ischaemic infarcts often associated with antiphospholipid antibodies.

Cerebral infarction

Computed tomography (CT)
- May not show infarction within 3 hours
- Majority will be abnormal within 2 to 4 days of symptom onset.
- Likely to miss small vessel lesions.

Magnetic resonance imaging (MRI)
- Should perform if CT normal.
- Sensitive to oedema
- More sensitive to the early stages of infarct (94%) specificity (100%)
- Multiple small vessel lesions seen as white hyperintense lesions representing thrombotic angiopathy (less often vasculitis in context of APS).
- Lesions not be specific to APS, e.g. found in normal ageing population.

Transcranial Doppler sonography—experimental
- Detects microembolic signals in blood vessels, not structural changes.
- May be predictive for future cardiovascular events in patients with internal carotid stenosis.
- High sensitivity, specificity in animal models.
- Reported to be useful in monitoring patients undergoing thrombolysis.

Neurocognitive dysfunction

Patients may present with poor attention, concentration, memory, fluency and psychomotor speed.

Magnetic resonance imaging (MRI)
- Cognitive symptoms do not correlate with MRI changes.

Positron emission tomography (PET)
- Impaired glucose metabolism may indicate altered cerebral perfusion but has not been well studied.

SPECT (single photon emission CT)
- May show hypoperfusion, research tool.

Chorea

This is a rare feature of APS; a review of 50 cases in APS demonstrated cerebral infarcts in only 35% on CT or MRI. PET scanning maybe useful in patients with negative MRI scans, sequential PET scans in two women with APS and chorea revealed striatal hypermetabolism.

Cerebral venous thrombosis

Patients present at a younger age with more extensive involvement than non-APS patients.

Headache present in 80% but may mimic many neurological conditions such as, meningitis, encephalopathy, benign intracranial hypertension (commonly), and stroke.

Magnetic resonance angiography (MRA)
- Investigation of choice largely replacing conventional angiography.

Transverse myelitis
MRI
- Investigation of choice
- Maybe normal in up to 30% scans even in classically presenting patients with SLE patients (usual associated with aPL).
- It has been reported that optic neuropathy occurs in up to 21% so opthalmological evaluation may be indicative.

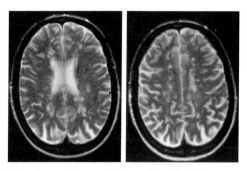

Fig. 11.12 Hyperintense white matter lesions on T2-weighted MRI.
Reproduced from Isenberg D and Renton P (eds) (2003). *Imaging in Rheumatology*. Oxford: Oxford University Press.

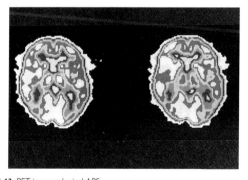

Fig. 11.13 PET in neurological APS.
Reproduced from Isenberg D and Renton P (eds) (2003). *Imaging in Rheumatology*. Oxford: Oxford University Press.

Cardiovascular imaging

Valvular heart disease

Valvular abnormalities are found in over a third of patients, mostly regurgitation of the mitral valve. Severe dysfunction occurs in 6% cases, half of these require replacement.

Antibiotic prophylaxis maybe advised prior to invasive procedures, although a surprisingly low incidence of infective endocarditis has been reported.

Transthoracic echocardiography
- Ideally all patients at diagnosis should have an echo.
- Indicated in cerebrovascular APS to look for aortic disease or intracardiac thrombosis.
- Transoesophageal echo (TOE) should be considered in cases of recurrent disease allowing more accurate diagnosis of infective vegetations and left-sided cardiac thrombi.

Ischaemic heart disease

A high aACL is an independent risk factor for myocardial infarction and recurrence rates are high.

Morphology of atherosclerotic coronary narrowing is the same as for non-APS patients and should be investigated in the same way, e.g. angiography.

Renal imaging

The renal vasculature may be involved in APS from the large vessels to the microvasculature mimicking glomerulonephritis.

Renal artery thrombosis

This is rare but may present as acute loin pain, systemic hypertension, haematuria, and renal failure.

Spiral CT
- Allows accurate diagnosis and attempts at revascularization.

Arteriography
- The gold standard
- Avoid unless active therapeutic intervention is being considered.

Renal venous thrombosis

This typically presents with acute loin pain and proteinuria.

Angiography
- The gold standard.

Spiral CT or MRA
- More commonly used for diagnosis, they are more specific than US.

Ultrasound
- High incidence of false negatives.
- May show increased renal size, altered echogenicity, loss of the corticomedullary junction, enlargement of the renal vein, possibly the thrombus.
- Better at showing thrombosis in transplanted kidneys which lie anteriorly.

Renal artery stenosis
Presents with moderate to severe hypertension, proteinuria and progressive renal impairment possibly with atherosclerotic disease elsewhere.

MRA (with gadolinium)
- Sensitivity 93–100%, specificity up to 98% for the main renal arteries.
- May miss distal renal artery and accessory artery lesions.

CT angiography
- No diagnostic benefits over MRA.
- Risks of potentially nephrotoxic contrast.

Angiography
- The gold standard.
- Allows therapeutic intervention, e.g. stenting or angioplasty.

ACE inhibitor scintigraphy
- May accurately assess the haemodynamic consequences of stenosis and act as a baseline prior to revascularization.

Thrombotic microangiopathy
This may cause a wide spectrum of severity of renal failure with proteinuria in primary APS thus is difficult to differentiate from SLE lupus nephritis, renal biopsy is required to make the diagnosis.

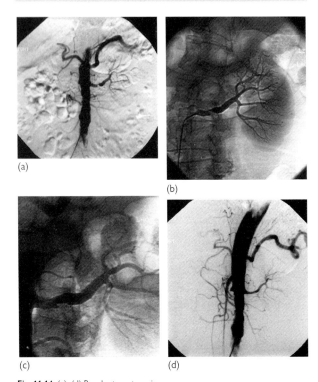

Fig. 11.14 (a)–(d) Renal artery stenosis.

Reproduced from Isenberg D and Renton P (eds) (2003). *Imaging in Rheumatology.*
Oxford: Oxford University Press.

Gastrointestinal imaging

Hepatic vein thrombosis
APS explains 20% of non-malignant cases of hepatic vein thrombosis.

Ultrasound
- Confirms diagnosis in 75% cases
- Improved by use of pulsed and colour Doppler.

Computed tomogrphy (CT)
- Useful when US shows non-specific changes.

Magnetic resonance imaging (MRI)
- Better IVC visualization.

Angiography
- Used when non-invasive tests are non-diagnostic, performed by direct transhepatic needle puncture of hepatic vein or retrograde cannulation of the superior vena cava (SVC) or inferior vena cava (IVC).

Acute intestinal infarction
APS may cause infarction and present as an acute abdomen, investigated as for non-APS patients, often diagnosed at laparotomy or on histology.

If chronic intestinal ischaemia occurs, intestinal angina may be diagnosed by angiography.

Opthalmological involvement

Classical cerebrovascular disease may present as amaurosis fugax or visual field defects, retinal artery or venous thrombosis which is picked up on fundoscopy, confirmed by fluorescein angiography.

▶ Optic neuropathy may be associated with nervous system pathology, e.g. transverse myelits, so it is advisable to perform MRI of the brain/spine in such patients.

Obstetric complications

During pregnancy all women with APS should be closely monitored by a multidisciplinary team including midwife, obstetrician, haematologist, rheumatologist. The use of low-dose aspirin and subcutaneous heparin have improved the live birth rate from 19 to 70%.

Ultrasound (US)
- Uterine artery Doppler waveform assessment should be performed in addition to routine US screening.
- High impedance waveforms with dichrotic notch is highly predictive of intrauterine growth factor (IUGR), pre-eclampsia, and placental abruption, poor foetal outcome

Systemic vasculitis

Introduction

Vasculitis is a rare condition characterized by blood vessel inflammation which can lead to aneurysm, stenosis causing ischaemic organ damage. This can be secondary e.g. to infection, malignancy, drug reactions or autoimmune rheumatic disease or primary.

The 1993 Chapel Hill classification of primary vasculitides uses the size of vessel involved, histopathology of lesions and clinical symptoms but is imperfect as some patients can not be classified or fit into more than one group.

Role of imaging

In practice, modern imaging has an important role in establishing a diagnosis by demonstrating (1) luminal changes, e.g. stenosis, occlusion, aneurysm (e.g. angiography in large/medium vessels); (2) inflammatory effects in organs.

MRA or contrast-enhanced CT may show vessel wall oedema and thickening of active vasculitis, PET, high resolution US maybe useful.

Large vessel vasculitis

Giant cell arteritis (GCA)

- Most common granulomatous large vessel vasculitis in the Caucasian population, rare under 50yrs age, predilection for temporal arteries.
- Classically presents with temporal headache, jaw claudication, often with malaise, weight loss, fever, polymyalgic symptoms, tenderness of the temples but irreversible blindness is the most feared complication.
- Imaging techniques are being evaluated which may avoid the need for biopsy which is itself problematic due to skip lesions (see Table 11.8).

Takayasu's arteritis (TA) (see Fig.11.15)

- Young women mostly affected(15–45yrs) in South East Asia/India.
- Involves the aorta (abdominal 50–60%), its branches (superior/inferior mesenteric 10–15%) and pulmonary arteries (50%).
- Early symptoms include non-specific malaise with markedly raised inflammatory markers.
- Later, limb claudication, intermittent or fluctuating visual loss, heart failure, pulmonary hypertension, or neurological problems with renovascular hypertension (the main cause of death).
- On examination, arterial pulses may be absent or decreased ('pulseless disease').

Table 11.8 Imaging methods to diagnose GCA/Takayasu's arteritis

Ultrasound	CT/MRA	PET	Arteriography*	
Site	Temporal artery	Extratemporal	Extratemporal	Extratemporal
Appearance	Hypoechoic halo[†]	↑ Gallium-67 uptake	↑ FDG-18 uptake	Smooth tapered stenosis
collaterals[‡]	e.g subclavian, axillary, brachial arteries			
Occlusions/stenosis	+	++	++	++
Aneursym (uncommon)	++	+		
Vessel wall inflammation	+	++	++	
Sensitivity	71–86%	MR[§] 80.6%	56%	
Specificity	93–100%	MR[§] 97%	98%	
Positive predictive value	50–84%	93%		
Negative predictive value	96–97.6%	80%		

*Or IV digital subtraction angiography (IV DSA). May distinguish pulmonary arteritis from embolism in TA.

[†]Perilumінal, should be seen in two planes to show circumferential halo due to oedema and stenosis. May guide biopsy site.

[‡]From external to internal carotid artery.

[§]High-resolution MRI.

Gallium-67 uptake decreases during remission, i.e. shows disease activity.

FDG-18 uptake in thoracic vessels most specific. Does not show isolated temporal involvement.

Occlusions/stenosis often bilateral, less often lower limbs.

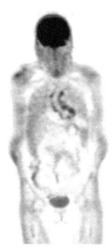

Fig. 11.15 Fludeoxyglucose (FDG) PET of TA (increased aortic uptake).
Reproduced from Isenberg D and Renton P (eds) (2003). *Imaging in Rheumatology.*
Oxford: Oxford University Press.

Medium vessel vasculitis

Polyarteritis nodosa (Pan)

- Necrotizing vasculitis of any medium/small artery, no glomerulonephritis.
- 10–20% associated with hepatitis B infection.
- The mean age of onset is 45–55yrs age, but can present at any age.
- Presents with malaise, weakness, weight loss, neuropathies, arthralgia, may involve the heart and cause vascular nephropathy.
- 60–80% gastrointestinal symptoms, 10–30% severe small bowel ischaemia and/or perforation, vessel aneurysms may rupture causing severe intra- and/or retroperitoneal bleeding.
- Small peripheral cerebral cortical and subcortical infarctions maybe seen.
- Visceral angiography shows stenosis/microaneurysm in 60–80% of cases.

Kawasaki disease

- Predominantly a disease of early childhood, highest incidence in Japan.
- Presents with fever, polymorphous exanthema on the palms/soles, reddening of the lips/mouth, bilateral conjunctivitis, cervical lymphadenopathy.
- One-third develop coronary artery vasculitis, one-third myocarditis.
- Aneurysms can develop (15–25%) which may resolve spontaneously or persist and progress to obstructive lesions causing myocardial infarction.
- Extra-coronary vascular lesions, e.g. renal, brachial or femoral artery aneurysms maybe seen more than a year after the acute presentation, particularly in the presence of giant aneurysms.

Transthoracic echocardiography (echo)

- Pericardial effusions in a third of cases.

Angiography

Ectasia (enlarged coronary arteries) or aneurysms (saccular/fusiform) maybe seen. High resolution cardiac US may also be helpful.

Small vessel vasculitis

This group includes anti-neutrophil cytoplasmic antibodies (ANCA)-associated vasculitides, e.g. Wegener's granulomatosis (WG), microscopic polyangiitis (MPA), Churg–Strauss syndrome (CSS) and non-ANCA associated (see Table 11.9).

Indium-11-labelled leucocyte scans

- May help to differentiate between WG and MPA, the latter does not show nasal uptake (more sensitive than X-ray)
- Both cause higher pulmonary uptake than controls and possibly splenic and gut abnormalities

Not sensitive in detecting renal vasculitis.

Table 11.9 Imaging of respiratory tract in ANCA-associated vasculitis

	Wegeners granulomatosis	Microscopic poylangitis	Churg–Strauss syndrome
Systems			
Upper respiratory	++	–	+
Lower respiratory	++	+	++
Ear nose throat	++	–	++
Ocular	+		–
Nervous system	+		++
Renal	++	++	++
Cardiac	++		
Gut			
Granuloma on biopsy	++	–	+/–
Chest X-ray			
Nodules	Bilateral>unilateral	Chronic (1–3mm on CT)	Reticulonodular opacities
Consolidation	Patchy or diffuse spares periphery	Bilateral, multifocal, peripheral/lobular	
	/apices, due to haemorrhage	due to haemorrhage	
Cavitating lesion	Common (50%)*	Rare	
	Pulmonary oedema	Bilateral hilar lymphadenopathy	
HRCT†	Interstitial lung disease	Acute bilateral consolidation	Bilateral patchy ground glass—lower zone

Table 11.9 (*Contd.*)

CT	Tracheobronchial lesions[‡]	Acute ground glass opacities	Halo sign surrounding consolidation/nodule[§]
	Nasal lesions (bone/septal erosion)	Pleural effusions 15%	
	Orbital lesions	Pulmonary oedema 6%	Bronchial wall thickening[i]

[*]Cavitating lesions have thick walls and irregular inner borders, may evolve to thin walled cysts or disappear with treatment.

[†]Recommended for evaluation of patients with WG to detect interstitial lung disease which maybe asymptomatic.

[‡]Tracheobronchial lesions such as focal or elongated stenosis, intra- or extraluminal soft tissue masses or thickening.

[$]The CXR evolves to show a reticular pattern in 2 to 3 days as blood absorbed into the interstitium and normalizes in 2 to 3 weeks if resolution occurs but if not then interstitial fibrosis may occur.

Any of these vasculitides can cause pleural effusions.

CT

[§]The halo of ground-glass opacity represents interstitial infiltration of eosinophils and giant cells surrounding a central core of haemorrhagic necrosis and granuloma.

[i]This can specifically distinguish CSS from other causes of eosinophilic pulmonary infiltrates.

Pulmonary angiography may distinguish arteritis from pulmonary embolism.

Wegener's granulomatosis (see Fig. 11.16)

- Triad of granulomatous inflammation of the respiratory tract, systemic vasculitis, and necrotizing crescentic vasculitis.
- Early symptoms can include chronic rhinitis, sinusitis or otitis.
- Peak incidence is at 40–50yrs age but can occur at any age, no gender predisposition.
- Biopsy of involved tissue is necessary to demonstrate necrosis and granulomatous inflammation, e.g. of nose/sinus, renal biopsies.

Microscopic polyangiitis

- Medium/small vessel vasculitis characterized by necrotizing and/or crescentic glomerulonephritis.
- Differs from WG because granulomas are not found and there is no ear nose or throat (ENT) or upper respiratory involvement.
- May present with fever, malaise, weight loss, arthralgias and purpura.
- Up to two-thirds have haemoptysis with or without alveolar or diffuse pulmonary haemorrhage.
- Renal impairment with proteinuria and microscopic haematuria are seen, most patients have rapidly progressive glomerulonephritis and may require dialysis.

Churg–Strauss syndrome

- Necrotizing vasculitis with eosinophilic infiltrates, occasionally granulomas.
- Peak incidence in third/fourth decade but can occur at any age.

- Vasculitic phase may present with malaise, weight loss, fever, muscle weakness, arthralgia, purpura, nodular skin lesions, abdominal pain, pericarditis, glomerulonephritis.
- Painful peripheral neuropathy may occur in more than two- thirds of cases with mononeuritis multiplex or symmetrical polyneuropathy.
- Prior to this a prodromal phase is common with allergic or eosinophilic infiltrative disease up to years before with rhinorrhoea, nasal polyps, recurrent sinusitis, and adult onset asthma.

Henoch–Schönlein purpura (HSP)

- Predominantly presenting in childhood, mean age of onset is 4 years.
- Typically presents with palpable purpura on the buttocks and extensor surfaces of the legs with lower limb oedema often preceded by an upper respiratory tract infection.
- Patients can also have colicky abdominal pain, vomiting, bloody diarrhoea, melaena, macroscopic haematuria, arthralgia/arthritis of the knees/ankles.

CT may show heterogeneous small bowel wall thickening (US will also), ascites, luminal narrowing and circular fold thickening.

Arteriography shows no abnormalities.

Rarely HSP is complicated by encephalopathy/CNS symptoms when MRI may show reversible changes in the white and grey matter.

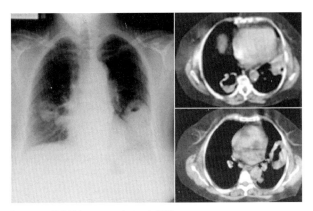

Fig. 11.16 CXR/CT—cavitating lesions in WG.
Reproduced from Isenberg D and Renton P (eds) (2003). *Imaging in Rheumatology*. Oxford: Oxford University Press.

Mixed essential cryoglobulinaemic vasculitis
- Cryoglobulinaemia may occur in isolation or secondary to haematological malignancy, infections, hepatitis C, autoimmune rheumatic diseases.
- Preferential involvement of venules, capillaries, and arterioles causing purpura, arthralgia and nephritis, less often alveolar haemorrhage.

Behçet's disease
- Classically causes orogenital ulceration and relapsing uveitis.
- May cause venothromboembolism, skin lesions, e.g. erythema nodosum.
- Pulmonary aneurysms may rupture and are a leading cause of death.

Pulmonary imaging, e.g. CXR/CT maybe abnormal, CT or MRI angiography maybe needed to differentiate pulmonary embolism from pulmonary arteritis complicated by thrombosis.

Isolated central nervous system angiitis
Limited to the central nervous system (CNS) often with a global dysfunction, e.g. headache, confusion, in one-third cranial neuropathies are seen. Biopsy is the gold standard for making the diagnosis, showing segmental granulmatous lesions.

Cerebral angiography
Not sensitive and can be normal because affected vessels are small but may show non-specific changes, e.g. multifocal/segmental narrowing, occlusion or microaneurysms, delayed emptying of vessels.

CT
May show non-specific changes.

MRI
Has a low specificity/sensitivity but may show white matter or subcortical disease and allow monitoring of response to therapy.

Imaging in bone and miscellaneous diseases

Osteoporosis

Osteoporosis is the commonest of the metabolic bone diseases, and is characterized by low bone masstt and an increase in fracture risk. Osteoporosis is silent until a fracture is sustained.

Clinical features

- Low trauma fractures are the hallmark of osteoporosis, with the commonest fractures being vertebral, hip, and wrist.
- The pain resulting from vertebral fracture may be minor and therefore dismissed by the patient. However, pain can be severe in a minority of cases.
- The natural history of vertebral fractures is of improvement of acute pain after approximately 6 weeks.
- Vertebral fractures are often associated with long-term pain and multiple fractures result in kyphosis and deformity.
- A rare but important complication of vertebral fracture is compression of the spinal cord.
- 20% of patients with hip fracture do not survive the next 12 months and in those that do, long-term care is often necessary.

Imaging modalities

Radiology

- Plain radiographs are useful in determining the outline and height of vertebral bodies, but do not determine the age of a fracture and are insensitive at detecting underlying bone pathology.
- Fractures of vertebral bodies commonly involve the anterior vertebral surface, with collapse of the upper end plate. The vertebral body may implode and sclerosis may be seen some weeks after the acute fracture reflecting either necrosis or trabecular compression.
- Less commonly posterior vertebral collapse may occur and retropulsion of the vertebral body may result in spinal cord compression.

▶ Plain radiographs remain the standard method for detecting fractures of long bones and MRI is often indicated in patients with vertebral fractures in detecting underlying pathology or when it is clinically useful to determine if a fracture is recent (see Fig. 12.1).

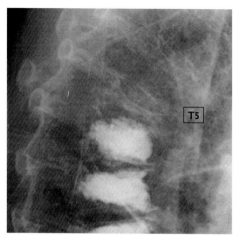

Fig. 12.1 Lateral plain film of the upper thoracic spine demonstrating a severe T5 vertebral compression fracture. Vertebroplasty cement is seen in the T6–T8 vertebrae.

DEXA

- Low bone densitometry indicates a risk of future fracture and is measured by dual X-ray absorptiometry (DEXA), a technique in which the radiation exposure is lower than that of daily background radiation.
- DEXA measures bone mineral density which is compared with peak bone mass (T score) and age matched bone mass (Z score) in a population cohort.
- The World Health Organisation definition of osteoporosis is 2.5 standard deviations below peak bone mass. Osteopaenia is defined as 1 standard deviation below peak bone mass and also carries an increased although less significant fracture risk. It is estimated that each reduction of one standard deviation below age-matched bone mass carries an increased fracture risk of two- to threefold.
- The need for repeat bone densitometry is yet to be fully established and therefore remains controversial. It is rarely indicated at intervals less than two years and usually only in patients on high-dose corticosteroid therapy.
- Bone density is only one predictor of fracture risk, and algorithms which recognize risk factors such as age, history of maternal fracture and predisposing comorbidities will become used in standard assessment of patients with osteoporosis.

▶ An increase in bone densitometry in the spine may reflect a therapeutic response but may also reflect trabecular compression due to vertebral fractures so assessment of the clinical situation is imperative (see Fig. 12.2).

Vertebral morphometry

- This technique is now widely available on modern DEXA scanners and provides accurate vertebral body height measurements, and has a lower radiation exposure than plain radiographs of the spine.

However, vertebral morphometry does not provide detail of underlying bone structure.

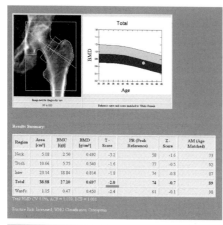

Reference curve and scores matched to White Female

Results Summary:

Region	Area [cm²]	BMC [(g)]	BMD [g/cm²]	T - Score	PR (Peak Reference)	Z - Score	AM (Age Matched)
Neck	5.08	2.50	0.492	-3.2	58	-1.6	73
Troch	10.66	5.75	0.540	-1.6	77	-0.5	92
Inter	23.14	18.84	0.814	-1.8	74	-0.8	87
Total	38.88	27.10	0.697	-2.0	74	-0.7	89
Ward's	1.05	0.47	0.450	-2.4	61	-0.1	98

Total BMD CV 1.0%, ACF = 1.039, BCF = 1.001

Fracture Risk: Increased, WHO Classification: Osteopenia

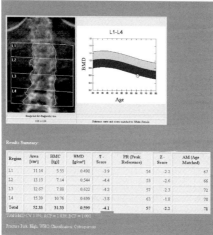

Reference curve and scores matched to White Female

Results Summary:

Region	Area [cm²]	BMC [(g)]	BMD [g/cm²]	T - Score	PR (Peak Reference)	Z - Score	AM (Age Matched)
L1	11.14	5.55	0.498	-3.9	54	-2.2	67
L2	13.13	7.14	0.544	-4.4	53	-2.6	66
L3	12.67	7.88	0.622	-4.2	57	-2.3	72
L4	15.39	10.76	0.699	-3.8	63	-1.8	78
Total	52.33	31.33	0.599	-4.1	57	-2.2	71

Total BMD CV 1.0%, ACF = 1.039, BCF = 1.001

Fracture Risk: High, WHO Classification: Osteoporosis

Fig. 12.2 Bone densitometry examination demonstrating bone mineral density measurements in the left hip and lumbar spine within the osteoporotic range (2 and 4.1 standard deviations below the average peak bone mass).

Magnetic resonance imaging (MRI)

- MRI is the imaging technique of choice in refractory back pain, as recommended by the Royal College of Radiology guidelines published in 2007.
- MRI provides detailed anatomy of both soft tissue and bone and infiltrative processes such as malignancy are detected more readily and earlier than on plain films. Soft-tissue changes of marrow metastases are seen as low signal areas on T1-weighted sequences.
- Marrow sensitive sequences (T2-weighted fat-suppression/STIR) show bone marrow oedema within acutely fractured vertebrae but is not commonly seen in more chronically fractured vertebrae.
- The pain of acute vertebral fracture usually settles within a few weeks, but where there is clinical doubt about the diagnosis, MRI maybe useful diagnostically.
- Identifying those patients with vertebral fracture, severe refractory pain and bone marrow oedema is useful clinically as this patient group may be suitable for vertebroplasy, in which bone cement is injected percutaneously into the collapsed vertebral body to stabilize the fracture and improve pain. Vertebroplasty can be undertaken at more than one level in patients with multiple fractures.
- MRI is also the most appropriate technique for evaluating canal dimensions in patients with acute fracture who are at risk of spinal cord compression and is mandatory in patients with neurological symptoms or signs.

▶ MRI is useful in determining detailed bone and soft tissue anatomy and detects oedema which characterizes acute osteoporotic vertebral compression fractures (Fig. 12.3).

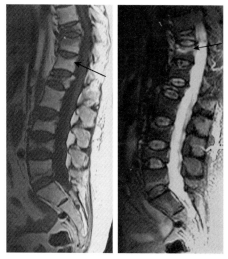

Fig. 12.3 MRI lumbar spine (T1-weighting and STIR sequences) showing multiple acute and chronic osteoporotic vertebral compression fractures.

Paget's disease

Paget's disease of bone is characterized by focal excessive bone resorption with a coupled excessive bone formation, and is of unknown aetiology.

Clinical features

- Symptoms vary depending on the site, extent and number of sites of skeletal involvement.
- Pain is the usual presenting feature in uncomplicated disease although asymptomatic disease may be picked up as an incidental finding on plain radiographs.
- The commonest bones affected include the bones of the pelvis, femur, tibia, humerus, vertebrae, and skull.
- Deformity is most obvious in individuals with long bone involement.
- Complications of Paget's disease include pathological fracture through abnormal bone, and pain arising from compression of local tissue such as nerve compression.
- Pain may also arise from joints which have developed osteoarthritis secondary to the altered mechanical stresses of adjacent deformed Pagetic bone.
- In fewer than 1% of patients, sarcomatous change may develop. It is more likely to occur in patients with widespread, or polystotic disease than those with monostotic disease.

Imaging modalities

Radiography

Plain radiographic appearances of Paget's disease (see Fig. 12.4)

The radiographic findings reflect the broad histopathological processes of Paget's disease.

- The first, or osteolytic phase, is characterized by rapid and extensive bone resorption by abnormal multinucleated osteoclasts and appears on plain radiographs as lucent areas or areas of osteolysis in the subarticular regions of long bones. This may extend to the diaphysis of an affected long bone, giving the radiological appearance of a wedge-shaped or flame-shaped lucency with clear demarcation from the adjacent normal bone.
- Coarsening of the trabeculae with bone expansion and underlying or adjacent lytic areas characterizes the second phase of Paget's disease which histopathologically combines excessive bone formation and osteolysis.
- The third phase reflects long-standing disease, which is usually inactive and which has no osteolytic areas, but sclerotic, thickened trabeculae. Bone bowing and pseudofractures may be present.

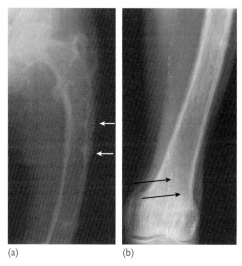

(a)   (b)

Fig. 12.4 Paget's disease. Plain films demonstrating (a) the chronic phase of Paget's disease (bone expansion and remodelling—bowing—with coarsened disorganized trabeculae and incremental fractures on the outer convex cortex) and (b) the active phase more distally (flame-shaped lucency pointing to the distal joint).

Long bones

- Deformity, bowing and secondary degenerative change in adjacent joints are detected on plain radiographs of long bones such as the femur and tibia.
- Fractures most commonly affect the femur and are seen distal to the lesser trochanter. Although they may progress to complete fractures, the commonest appearance is of incomplete fractures, sometimes multiple, and perpendicular to the cortex on the convexity of the bowed long bone.

Skull

- Osteolytic areas in the skull are seen in early disease and indicate areas of bone resorption in the inner and outer tables of the skull. The term osteoporosis circumscripta is used to describe this appearance.
- A cotton wool appearance of patchy new bone formation may be seen in later disease.
- Involvement of the outer table leads to generalized bony expansion of the skull and can occur with or without osteoporosis circumscripta.
- Patients with skull involvement may develop basilar invagination which arises as a result of remodeling of soft bone and appears on plain images as intracranial displacement of the foramen magnum (Tam O'Shanter appearance).

Osteosarcoma

Osteosarcoma is a rare complication of Paget's disease and may be difficult to diagnosis clinically and radiologically, but may appear radiologically as an expanding bony mass.

Isotope bone scan

Isotope bone scans are useful in determining the extent of disease, which may not be clinically obvious, but important in clinical management when monitoring for complications of the disease.

Computed tomography (CT) and magentic resonance imaging (MRI)

These are useful techniques for determining nerve compression, for example in patients with symptoms or signs of cranial nerve or spinal cord compression, and for patients with symptomatic basilar invagination. CT and MRI are also used in staging patients with osteosarcoma.

▶ MRI and CT are useful techniques in patients with neurological complications.

Complex regional pain syndrome

Complex regional pain syndrome (CRPS) Type 1 is the preferred term for this syndrome which has been previously called algodystrophy, RSD (reflex sympathetic dystrophy), and Sudek's atrophy, amongst others. CRPS type 2 is reserved for those patients with associated nerve injury.

Clinical features

- In the majority of cases there is a history of trauma, fracture or recent surgery. However, CRPS can also occur in association with non-traumatic disease, e.g. radicular pain and with no predisposing factors.
- The symptoms comprise severe pain, with sensory, vasomotor, sudomotor, and motor involvement.
- Unilateral symptoms are usual although bilateral symptoms are reported.
- Sensory changes are evident, and in particular hyperalgesia. Alteration in temperature or skin colour, oedema and motor dysfunction are characteristic.

Stages

Three stages are recognized, although the natural history remains unclear.

- The first is the acute/warm stage where there is acute onset of pain, with warmth, oedema, and swelling of the affected area.
- The second phase reflects more established disease and is characterized by cyanosis, coldness and muscle wasting but without oedema.
- The third stage is atrophic with less pain and swelling but with a poor functional outcome and prognosis.

Imaging modalities

Radiography

- Localized osteopaenia, indicating bone loss of at least 30%, may be obvious when plain radiographs of the affected side are compared with the unaffected side.
- Patchy loss occurs early and the appearance becomes more diffuse in late disease.

▶ Normal plain films do not exclude a diagnosis of RSD as the diagnosis is made clinically.

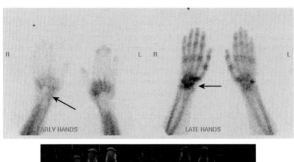

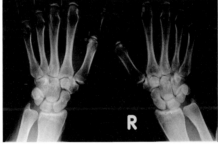

Fig. 12.5 Radionuclide bone scan demonstrating reduced blood flow in the right wrist in the early blood pool phase and diffusely increased bone activity (increased tracer uptake) in the late bone phase consistent with a diagnosis of complex regional pain syndrome (reflex sympathetic dystrophy). The corresponding plain film demonstrates global demineralization of the right carpus.

Magnetic resonance imaging (MRI)

- The MRI findings in CRPS are non-specific and include soft-tissue swelling, soft tissue and bone oedema best seen with a fat-suppressed T2-weighted sequence, and is a valuable technique in excluding other pathologies.
- Soft tissue oedema is only seen in patients with early, warm CRPS and is not demonstrated in patients with later, cold disease.
- There are other conditions which may present in a similar way clinically but which have different radiological appearances. These are:
  - Transient osteoporosis, a syndrome characterized by acute onset of pain and radiographic evidence of localized osteoporosis. The proximal femur is the site most commonly involved, resulting in the term transient osteoporosis of the hip, which is associated with pregnancy. Symptoms may last as long as 2 years but may respond to bisphosphonate therapy or drilling the bone. The relationship of transient osteoporosis to CRPS is yet to be established and understood.
  - Transient bone marrow oedema syndrome, also of unknown aetiology, differs from transient osteoporosis as there is no evidence of osteopenia on plain radiographs although bone marrow oedema is present on MRI. Symptoms are generally self-limiting, and it is possible that a spectrum of disease, from bone marrow oedema through to stage 3 CRPS, exists.

Other imaging modalities

Isotope bone scintigraphy

- Three-phase bone scintigraphy reveals a typical pattern of increased blood flow and soft tissue uptake in the early, blood pool phase of the scan, and increased bone uptake at 3–4 hours. However, in stage 3, the changes are indistinguishable from those seen in chronic disuse syndrome.

Three-phase bone scintigraphy is not routinely performed but is indicated if CRPS is suspected.

Heritable disorders of the skeleton

Hereditable musculoskeletal conditions include those which affect bone and cartilage such as osteopetrosis and chondroplasias, and those conditions which affect collagen, such as Marfan's syndrome and Ehlers–Danlos syndrome.

Osteopetrosis

- Osteopetrosis or marble bone disease is a rare condition in which there is a marked increase in bone density due to an accumulation of bone which has not been resorbed because of abnormal osteoclast function.
- Both autosomal dominant and autosomal recessive forms are recognized, the former often picked up incidentally but the later resulting in premature death unless diagnosed and treated at an early stage.
- The clinical features are of excessively dense brittle long bones which fracture with minor trauma.

Imaging modalities

Radiography

- Plain radiographs are diagnostic in acute fractures, but may also reveal generalized increased bone density of cortical bone or sclerosis.
- Metaphyseal modeling is abnormal in osteopetrosis, with a club-shape within the long bones, where focal sclerosis displaces normal marrow, and is termed the 'bone in bone' appearance. (see Fig. 12.6).

Osteogenesis imperfecta

- Osteogenesis imperfecta, or brittle bone syndrome, is caused by mutations in type 1 collagen structural genes and causes a range of extraskeletal abnormalities, some of which result from bone fragility and increased risk of fracture and bone deformity. Four main types are recognised and vary in severity.
- Type 1 is the mildest variant, type 11 results in foetal death, type 111 and IV tend are severe and characterized by recurrent fractures and deformity.

Imaging modalities

Radiography

Plain radiographs may reveal generalized osteopenia and associated fractures involving the skull, chest, spine, limbs and pelvis, depending on the type and severity.

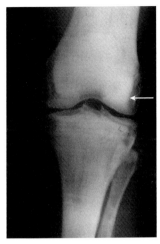

Fig. 12.6 Plain film demonstrating bony sclerosis and 'bone a bone' appearance in osteopetrosis representing a core of more primitive, abnormally formed endosteal ossification.

Marfan's syndrome (see Fig. 12.7)

- Marfan's syndrome is a multisystem disease which may involve the musculoskeletal, cardiovascular, ocular, and pulmonary systems, the skin and dura.
- It is caused by mutation of the fibrillin gene *FBN1*.
- To fulfil the diagnostic criteria, two different organ systems must be involved in addition to either a third system or a family history of the disease.
- Cardiovascular disease, either aortic root rupture or dissection, is the most common cause of premature death.
- Diagnosis is made clinically, although fibrillin mutation analysis is now available in some centres.

Imaging modalities

Radiography

- Scoliosis, spondylolisthesis and protrusio acetabuli are all features of Marfan's syndrome which may be detected with plain radiographs.
- Echocardiography is diagnostic in mitral valve prolapse and dilation of the aortic root and is indicated at regular intervals in monitoring cardiac disease.

Magnetic resonance imaging (MRI)

- Dural ectasia is detected on MRI of the spine where the pressure of CSF distends the abnormally thin dura.
- MRI is indicated in asymptomatic patients if the diagnosis of dural ectasia will confirm the diagnosis of Marfan's syndrome if insufficient organ involvement criteria have been met.

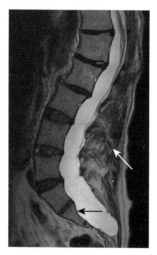

Fig. 12.7 MRI lumbar spine demonstrating dural ectasia with scalloping of the posterior vertebral body wall of the upper sacral segments in a patient with Marfan's disease.

Index